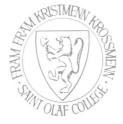

HIPPOCRATES NOW! IS YOUR DOCTOR ETHICAL?

Becoming an informed health care consumer is not always easy. Faced with advances in medical technology, and changing economic and social realities, it's sometimes difficult to know if the decisions you and your doctor are making are the best for you, and if they are in fact ethical.

Understanding how doctors make decisions, and knowing about the kinds of ethical dilemmas they face, are important, as is understanding how the health care systems in both the United States and Canada work. Any modern health care system, whether funded by the state, private insurance, or direct billing to patients, presents choices for both you and your doctor. You, the consumer, need to learn how to be your own advocate.

Hippocrates Now! helps guide you through aspects of health care that are clearly, and sometimes not so clearly, affected by the ethical conduct of both doctors and patients. The authors, an experienced medical writer/educator and a family physician, are in a unique position to examine these issues. They discuss the human fallibility of doctors and matters that concern everyone, for example, consent to medical treatment, confidentiality, patients' rights, and AIDS. These complex issues generate questions that demand complex answers. It is difficult, however, to communicate with your doctor about these issues if you speak a 'different language' and place different values on the same things. This book bridges the gap between you and your doctor. The authors teach you how to be better informed in order to maintain control of decisions that affect your health care, both now and in the future.

PATRICIA PARSONS is a professor of public relations at Mount Saint Vincent University and a medical writer.
ARTHUR PARSONS is a family physician and was Chairman of the Canadian Medical Association's Committee on Ethics for ten years.

PATRICIA PARSONS, B.N., M.Sc.
ARTHUR PARSONS, M.D.

Hippocrates Now!
Is Your Doctor Ethical?

UNIVERSITY OF TORONTO PRESS
Toronto Buffalo London

© Patricia Houlihan Parsons and Arthur H. Parsons 1995
Toronto Buffalo London
Printed in Canada

ISBN 0-8020-0526-8 (cloth)
ISBN 0-8020-6963-0 (paper)

Printed on acid-free paper

Canadian Cataloguing in Publication Data

Parsons, Arthur H. (Arthur Hedley), 1943–
  Hippocrates now! : Is your doctor ethical?

  Includes bibliographical references and index.
  ISBN 0-8020-0526-8 (bound) ISBN 0-8020-6963-0 (pbk.)

  1. Medical ethics, I. Parsons, Patricia Houlihan.
  II. Title.

  R724.P37 1995   174'.2   C94-932425-6

University of Toronto Press acknowledges the financial assistance to its
publishing program of the Canada Council and the Ontario Arts Council.

Contents

vi   Contents

PART III: The New Everyday Ethics

The Oath of Hippocrates

I swear by Apollo, the Physician, by Aesculapius, by Hygeia, by Panacea, by all the gods and goddesses, to keep, according to my ability and my judgement, the following Oath:

'To hold the one who taught me this art equally precious to me as my parents; to share my assets with him and, if need be, to see to his needs; to treat his children in the same manner as my brothers and to teach them this art free of charge or stipulation, if they desire to learn it; that by maxim, lecture and every other method of teaching, I will bestow a knowledge of the art to my own sons, to the sons of my teacher and to disciples who are bound by a contract and oath, according to the law of medicine and no one else; I will adhere to that method of treatment which, to the best of my ability and judgement, I consider beneficial for my patients and I will disavow whatever is harmful and illegal; I will administer no fatal medicine to anyone even if solicited, nor will I offer such advice; in addition, I will not provide a woman with an implement useful for abortion.

'I will live my life and practice my art with purity and reverence. I will not operate on someone who is suffering from a stone but will leave this to be done by those who perform such work. Whatever house I enter, I will go therein for the benefit of the sick and I will stand free from any voluntary criminal action and corrupt deed and the seduction of females or males, be they slaves or free. I will not divulge anything that, in connection with my profession or otherwise, I may see or hear of the lives of men which should not be revealed, on the belief that all such things should be kept secret.

'So long as I continue to be true to this Oath, may I be granted happiness of life, the practice of my art and the continuing respect of all men. But if I foreswear and violate this Oath, may my fate be the opposite.'

Before We Begin ...

Consider first the well-being of the patient ...
– Hippocrates

This book is for people who wouldn't normally pick up a book about medical ethics as well as for those who would. It is also for everyone else who cares about what is happening to the practice of medicine in North America today.

Hippocrates' instruction seems to be simple enough, but it has become increasingly complex in medical practice recently. Hippocrates, the acknowledged 'Father of Medicine,' believed passionately in making the patient the centre of all medical encounters. If a type of treatment is right for the patient, then it must be right. But Hippocrates hadn't bargained on artificial hearts, multi-organ transplants, fetal therapy, *in vitro* fertilization, MRIs, and the list of modern medical marvels that fill our North American hospitals. Nor did he bargain on the doctors who practise medicine today. Imagine what might happen if Hippocrates attended rounds in a sprawling inner-city hospital some morning; he would be astounded.

There has, however, been a renaissance of concern lately for what is ethical. After the hedonism of the 1970s and the materialism of the 1980s, according to the trend watchers the 1990s are the decade of ethics; everybody seems to have something to say about it. Lawyers are talking about ethical procedures in the courtroom; business magazines are talking about ethics in the business world; popular magazines are talking about sexual ethics; and even high school students are taking courses in ethics. It is hardly surprising, then, that currently one of the arenas in which ethics is being debated most heatedly is medicine and health care, where the decisions made relate directly to issues of life and death – the basic concerns that give most of us cause to pause and consider what is happening, at least from time to time.

With all of this discussion about ethics, one has to wonder if everyone reading the magazines, watching the television documentaries, and listening to the ethical debates really knows what ethics is. A medical ethics textbook would probably tell you that ethics is the systematic study of morality and concerns itself with the verification or validation of moral judgments. If that is the most salient definition of ethics available to the average consumer, why would so many people be concerned about, or even try to understand, ethics? The fact is that many people do not understand ethics, and those in the medical profession have done relatively little to help the average person to improve that understanding. The world of medical ethics is unlike that in which most of us live. It is full of 'shoulds' and 'oughts' and difficult questions with unclear answers. Medical ethicists, for all their contemplation of the issues, have not yet truly cracked that communication barrier which so often arises between those who know and those who do not. This is, however, to be expected, at least to some extent. Most of us rarely consider, at least overtly, the ethical implications of each of our actions. Medical ethicists, on the other hand, must consider the moral rightness or wrongness of each action they recommend. In doing so, they come face to face with life-and-death dramas at every turn. No doubt, this can be draining.

The problem with most of what we see in medical ethics today is that it seems so esoteric, concerned with big words to define moral principles. What most people really want to know is: how do these issues and judgments about what is right and wrong and whether something is really worthy of being done really affect me and my family? How does my doctor make his or her ethical decisions or, even more frightening, does my doctor even recognize an ethical problem when faced with one? Or does my doctor think that everything can be boiled down to a science?

Why is it that ethics in medicine and health care have become such popular topics among the general public? Why now? For centuries, physicians and others working in health care have grappled with life-and-death questions and made decisions about what was right or wrong, and they did this with essentially little input from those less knowledgeable about medicine itself. Why, then, do people now see the need to be involved in these decisions? And why have we seen the emergence of a new health-related occupation, that of the medical ethicist, a field recognized by academic institutions and the subject of new academic programs? There are far more questions than there are answers, but we will try to answer some.

Probably the most important factor contributing to this new awareness is the enormously powerful media portrayal of the new medical technologies. Every sensational case, every medical breakthrough, is front-page news. In addition, fictionalized portrayals of medical dilemmas ranging from transplant technology to genetic engineering have reached millions of people via television, novels, and movies.

Both something good and something bad have resulted from this media blitzing over the past decade or two. The good outcome is the thirst among the general population for more information about health care in general, and their own health care in particular. This heightened awareness has resulted in the sweeping consumerism that has made many people want more control over the decisions that affect them personally. The bad outcome is that most of the media coverage is of the more high-profile, high-tech side of medicine; as a result, the everyday, practical issues that affect everyone often seem to be lost in the shuffle. The significance of the dozens of decisions made daily by a family doctor in his or her office seems to pale in comparison with that of dramatic judgments dealing with life or death. The fact is that the decisions made every day in the family doctor's office are, indeed, related to life-and-death issues but their effects are unlikely to be as spectacular or as imminent.

Media coverage has taken medical ethics beyond the hospital and consulting room. We now hear about doctors going on strike; the widespread sexual abuse of patients; doctor-designed suicide machines; the unknowing and trusting patient who is inseminated with her doctor's own sperm in some kind of personal power trip; the doctor who, aware that he carries the hepatitis virus, continues to operate on patients and infects several; the view of medical societies that their members have no responsibility to inform a patient about their own HIV status; the confusion about doctors' relationships with drug companies.

As a result of this unprecedented interest in medical ethics as well as a clearer recognition of the fact that dilemmas do, indeed, exist, the medical ethicist was born. An ethicist is trained in the philosophical approach to making decisions about right and wrong, and frequently has no training in medical care. Thus, the physician and the ethicist afford us two different views of the world. These views, the esoteric and the practical, must be married and considered equally before well-thought-out, functional decisions can be made with us and for us. Philosophers interested in the moral decisions made by medical practitioners have been around for many years, but only recently have they been given a real role to play in our health-care system.

Today it is crucial for us to bring our expectations regarding health care in line with the realities of present-day economics and medical science. In this book, we will provide you with a view of medical ethics that you might not have considered. Its premise is that if you, the health care consumer, are better informed about issues and trends, you will become an active participant in making decisions, both large and small, that will affect your medical care and that of your family.

When you walk into your doctor's office, you are unaware of the moral judgments that he or she has been making that very day, even that very hour, and might have to make while you are seated in the office. Doctors are only human, and the sooner that you, as a consumer, realize not only the potential but also the limitations of the science of modern medicine and its providers, the sooner you will both understand the pressures and demand that you be given a larger role in the decision-making processes. Uninformed health care consumers, however, can do little that is of positive use in making these thorny decisions. Complex questions often demand complex answers, and it is difficult to communicate with our doctors about these issues when we speak a different language and place different values on the same things.

We will take you through the minefield of today's medical ethics by introducing you to the issues and concerns that affect each of us. We will make you privy to information that has been published in both the academic and the non-academic medical press. In other words, we will share with you some of the material that your doctor reads. We will also help you to develop some skills for becoming more involved in the decisions that will affect you personally. Finally, we will guide you through the dilemmas that may affect you indirectly now, but will have an impact on the future of health care for our children and their children. You owe it to yourself to take an active part in the ethical dilemmas that affect us all.

To return briefly to Hippocrates: the Hippocratic tradition of medical ethics may not be the most widely accepted today in medical circles, but his is the name that the layperson most closely associates with this field. Thus, *Hippocrates Now!* is the modern patient's look at ethics.

PHP & AHP

PART I

EVERYDAY MEDICAL ETHICS: ISSUES FOR EVERYONE

Most of us would probably find it difficult to think of one person we know who has never or will never have occasion to use the services of the medical care system on this continent. The majority of North Americans are born in hospitals and, in fact, also die in hospitals. In between, there can be any number of encounters with doctors. Thus, there are questions of medical ethics that affect every one of us.

Part I presents some of these issues, both those that are modern and those that have their beginnings in the history of medicine as it is practised in North America today. Here we offer you some information, some questions, and some suggestions about how to deal with these issues when they touch your life or the lives of your loved ones.

1
A Dilemma a Day

I will live my life and practice my art with purity and reverence ...
– The Oath of Hippocrates

Dr Barry Goode awoke from what seemed to have been just a short nap after delivering a healthy baby at 4:00 a.m. and readied himself for another day in his office. He had no reason to think that today would be very different from any other day, but he was still exhilarated at the thought of his work. At age forty-six, Dr Goode has been a family physician for twenty years. Considered to be at the prime of his career, he has a very busy general practice and prides himself on keeping his skills updated and constantly sharpened by participating in a variety of continuing education activities.

As Dr Goode walked into his office through his waiting-room that morning, he noted that it was full, and that there were several unfamiliar patients waiting to see him. He never ceased to marvel at the fact that, after twenty years of practising medicine in the same city, he was still receiving calls from people looking for a new doctor.

After he donned his white lab coat and stuffed a stethoscope, tongue depressors, and several lollipops in his pockets, he went into his examining-room and asked Susan, his nurse, to send in the first patient.

The first patient of the morning was Mrs Kendall, a fifty-year-old woman who had been coming to see Dr Goode for the past five years. She was in the office an average of three times a month, always with a different complaint. Dr Goode always investigated when he thought that there might be a problem, and listened patiently and reassuringly when that was what she needed. He occasionally felt frustrated by her complaints and by his frequent lack of success in 'fixing' them, but he tried not to show it. Today's visit was much the same as any other, but this time she was requesting a repeat mammogram (a breast X-ray). She had had her yearly mammogram six months earlier and she had no family history of breast cancer, and currently had no symptoms. A close friend, however, had recently been diagnosed with this disease. Dr Goode knew that, at present, there was a waiting-list for mammography. Should he call his friend, a radiologist at the local hospital, and ask him to squeeze this patient in because she is concerned, thereby displacing someone else on the waiting-list? He decided he would see what his partners thought about it, and put Mrs Kendall's chart aside for later.

His next patient was the fifteen-year-old daughter of a physician friend of his with whom he played bridge every Wednesday night. She was not sick, but she was asking him to prescribe the birth-control pill. And no, he could not breathe a word of this to her father. Should he prescribe medication to a minor without the knowledge and consent of her parents?

Mr Sampson was the next patient to enter his office that morning. A thirty-year-old married man, Mr Sampson was making a return visit to Dr Goode to discuss the results of the tests he had had done in the office the week before. Mr Sampson's test results indicated that he had a sexually transmitted disease. Dr Goode explained to him that the condition would be relatively easy to treat, but that he would have to tell his pregnant wife so that she too could be treated. Since Mr Sampson had contracted the disease from an extramarital source, he refused to let Dr Goode call his wife, and further refused to tell her himself. Should Dr Goode betray the confidence of his patient and tell his wife anyway? Should he call her obstetrician? Or should he put this woman, and perhaps her unborn child, at risk by his silence?

By lunch time, Dr Goode's mind was in a spin from all of the dilemmas he had faced in the morning. He looked at his calendar and noticed that he was scheduled to attend a staff meeting chaired by the manager of his and his partners' offices. He grabbed a sandwich and the morning paper, and went along to the meeting. Priding himself on being able to do several things at once, he ate, read the paper, and listened to the proceedings, all at the same time. Suddenly, he stopped eating and reading and began to listen more carefully. The office manager was reporting that the on-site laboratory's productivity for the month was down, and she was requesting that the physicians consider stepping up the number of lab tests that they were ordering. He couldn't believe his ears, and spoke up to ask if she was suggesting that they order unnecessary tests in an effort to increase revenue. Everyone in the room just looked at him.

When he returned to his office, his receptionist told him that the employer of one of his patients was on the telephone, waiting to speak with him. As he took the call, Dr Goode was thinking about how much simpler things had seemed in the early days of his practice. The caller was asking him about the medical condition of his employee, a man whose work entailed the use of very dangerous equipment. He was asking specific questions and demanding specific answers. While Dr Goode recognized the fact that this man felt he had a right to know about the sickness/ wellness of his employee, and the employee did, in fact, have a medical condition that would make his work even riskier, the patient had a right to privacy. Should he tell the man anything at all, or refuse to discuss it?

Dr Goode went home that day, realizing that this was just a typical day in the life of a family doctor.

- Should a physician ever order tests or treatment without medical indication, just because the patient wants it?
- Should patients be required to wait their turn for scarce medical care, or are there good reasons for 'bumping'? If there are good reasons, who should make this decision?
- Should a physician ever treat an underage child in a non-emergency situation without first getting parental consent?

- How can a physician decide which patient's rights should be upheld in a situation in which one patient's rights are in conflict with another's?
- Can a physician's desire to make money ever be allowed to compromise the quality of care he or she is giving a patient?
- Is there ever a good reason to breech patient confidentiality?

These constitute but a small sample of the ethical questions faced every day by the average physician in his or her office. They are hardly the stuff of a block-buster movie of the week or a best-selling novel. They are not all high-tech, and they are not all high-profile. But they are real, and they are frightening because their solutions frequently are left to one individual whose own values and personal ethics will often determine the course of action. Can you always trust this person to do the right thing? To be 'ethical'?

Before you can even begin to answer these questions, you need to know what ethics really is.

- ideals
- morals
- mores
- scruples
- standards

All of these words give some idea of what ethics is all about, but none of them really defines ethics in any useful way. One ancient Roman definition of ethics had this to say: 'Live uprightly, hurt no one, give to each his due.' This description still rings true today. Ethics is concerned with making decisions about right and wrong while assuring that everyone affected by those decisions is taken into consideration and not hurt. Trying to decide upon the best course of action in a given situation is confounded when rights come into conflict, when the likely results are not clear-cut, and when the outcome will be bad, regardless of which alternative is chosen. An ethical examination of a situation, then, helps us to determine how something worth doing might best be accomplished from the perspective of what is morally right or morally wrong.

THE HISTORICAL ROOTS OF MEDICAL ETHICS

Those practising medicine and other types of health care have been concerned for centuries about 'doing the right thing.' In the fourth century B.C., the profession took upon itself the task of adopting an oath that would set out its ideals, its promise to the world of how medicine would be practised. That, of course, is what we know today as the Hippocratic Oath, named for Hippocrates. Another of Hippocrates' contributions was his introduction of logic into the practice of medicine. He also considered the foremost characteristic of physicians to be not their ability to understand biochemistry, physics, or physiology, but their ethical behaviour.

Late in the twelfth century, a Spanish-born Hebrew philosopher called Maimonides examined science and medicine from a Jewish perspective. However, from the time of Hippocrates until the eighteenth century, little of how physicians felt about ethics in medicine seems to have had an impact on the way we think about ethics today.

Formalization of medical ethics is attributed to two Englishmen, John Gregory and Thomas Percival (Baker, Porter, and Porter 1993). Two of their important contributions are Gregory's *Lectures on the Duties and Qualifications of Physicians* (1772) and Percival's *Medical Ethics* (which first appeared in 1770 as *Observations on the Duties and Offices of a Physician*). The latter was evidently written as a set of rules to settle some kind of a dispute that had erupted in the Manchester Infirmary.

It was in the latter part of the eighteenth century that modern medical ethics began to emerge as the medical profession began organizing itself into associations, and thus political forces. The first discussions of medical ethics centred around what we today would simply call 'manners.' In 1849, the British Medical Association, which had been formed in 1832, appointed a committee on ethics and, two years later, a committee to develop a framework for a code of ethics. Shortly after that, both the American and Canadian Medical Associations developed their first codes of ethics to guide the practice of their members.

In an address to the medical graduates of Harvard University in 1858, which was revisited in a 1988 issue of a medical journal, physician-author Oliver Wendell Holmes spoke about moral duties of physicians: 'Your duty as physicians involves the practice of every virtue and the shunning of every vice' (Holmes 1988, 129). He went on to say that these neophyte doctors should be truthful, charitable, and respectful of their own profession.

Although physicians have always attempted to practise 'ethical' medicine, only in recent years have such enormous controversies developed in the field. Factors outside of the profession, such as consumer concern about the behaviour of professionals, media attention to both problems and successes in medicine, and the increasing size of the health care system, have contributed to this new interest in medical ethics. Similarly, within the profession, new medical and technological breakthroughs have caused doctors to change the way they view many different aspects of the human condition, and what is right and wrong.

THE ROOTS OF WHAT IS 'RIGHT'

One fact is clear: medical ethics is firmly rooted in the general morality of the society in which it is being examined. For example, in a society in which human life is believed to begin at the moment of conception, the decision to allow the development of abortion clinics is not an issue at all. There would be no discussion; they would not be tolerated. Clearly, then, an individual society's mores at a particular point in history play a major part in the development of ethical standards; thus, what is right and what is wrong can change over time.

If you are the average health care consumer, the one factor, above all others, that affects the decisions that will be made by your doctor is *who that doctor is*: where he or she came from, what kind of person the doctor is, and what values he or she has adopted. In other words, one of the most important factors which govern a doctor's medical-ethical decisions is what can be called 'personal ethics.' Personal ethics grow out of the values to which an individual is exposed throughout life, not just in medical school. These value systems go back to how that doctor was treated as a child and his or her personal experiences of growing up and view of the world. When the doctor's personal value system – which, like it or not, is frequently applied to professional situations – is not compatible with yours, the inevitable result is conflict.

In an attempt to avoid just that sort of personal bias entering into the process of making ethical decisions, doctors can rely on a series of ethical principles. Over the years, the medical profession has tried to define and refine this series of principles and to base decisions upon them. These principles can be viewed as laws, rules, or simple guidelines, depending upon your viewpoint. Despite the efforts of some medical licensing boards, no objective tribunal exists for judging whether or not such principles have been applied appropriately in each situation, nor is there an immediate penalty for failing to apply them appropriately. The processes within the self-governing medical profession for dealing with breaches in moral conduct are often long and cumbersome from the patient's point of view. In addition, some believe that the use of rules to make ethical decisions is too limiting and would prefer to rely upon the analysis of each individual situation at the time of occurrence, but more about that later.

The principles upon which ethical decisions have been based for many hundreds of years can be simple to understand – yes, simple to understand – but difficult to apply in real situations.

The first principle that has governed the ethical practice of medicine for many hundreds of years is the concept of *the sanctity of life*. In other words, life is precious and should be preserved. The application of this principle has gotten many a supporter of abortion-on-demand into ethically treacherous territory as society continues to grapple with the controversy over when the fetus is, in fact, a human life. Similarly, it is this principle which causes the conflict in the decision to terminate treatment for individuals with life-threatening illness, the decision that enough is enough. Some observers have said that practitioners of modern medicine have yet to learn that concept as they continually attempt to maintain some semblance of life at all costs. With modern medical technology, the problem has become defining life in the first place.

The second principle upon which the solution of some ethical dilemmas rests is that of *autonomy*. Autonomy is personal liberty. When physicians apply this concept, they consider that patients have a right to make their own decisions when given adequate information and that the patient is frequently the best judge of what direction his or her medical care should take. The idea that the patient should be more of a partner with the doctor, then, is not a new one. The last decade, however, has seen the rise of consumerism and demands for more control by the patient.

Applying the principle of autonomy helps the physician to help patients to help themselves. The opposite of autonomy is what is called *paternalism*. This, the 'all-knowing father' concept leads the physician, and indeed the health care system in general, to treat the patient much as one would a child. In applying it, the doctor believes he or she always knows what is best for the patient, and this way of thinking has contributed to many an ethical dilemma.

The third principle is that of *justice*. In applying it, the physician is guided to treat all patients as equals and to provide equivalent treatment for all who seek help for the same problem. This concept is sorely abused in instances where there simply is not enough to go around. For instance, when there are three suitable transplant candidates for a donor heart, how is the decision made to choose only one when all are deserving and all face death without that transplant? As the old saying goes, 'All men are created equal. Some are just more equal than others.'

The fourth principle goes back directly to the Hippocratic Oath; that is, *to do good* and *to do no harm*. (The philosophical terms for these are 'beneficence' and 'non-maleficence,' respectively). This principle speaks for itself, as it is the doctor's

responsibility to do the best for the patient under the circumstances and to avoid harming the patient. Following this rule
creates dilemmas when the treatment of the patient also has
harmful effects. For example, almost every time a physician
writes a prescription for a medication, he or she must weigh the
risks of that medication (every drug known to man has side-
effects for at least some patients) against its benefits. Usually,
the side-effects are so minimal, and the benefits so obvious, that
the dilemma never demands conscious resolution from a doctor,
but it is a consideration all the same. The real dilemma arises
when (a) the value of taking the drug or undergoing the treatment is equal to or less than the hazards involved, or (b) the seriousness of the problem has been overestimated. This situation is
aggravated by what doctors perceive as their need to protect
themselves against accusations of malpractice; doctors may
resort to overtreatment in an attempt to rationalize the exposure
of the patient to the risks of the medical treatment.

APPLYING THE PRINCIPLES

As we mentioned earlier, not everyone either in medicine or in
the field of medical ethics agrees with the 'rule-application'
approach. Some people prefer to assess each situation independently and not be bound by inflexible principles. This approach,
sometimes called 'situation ethics,' has grown in popularity in
recent years as it becomes more difficult to apply the laws
equally to everyone. Situation ethics creates a different problem
for the patient, who must try to decide whether or not to trust
the person who will make that decision without benefit of outside guidelines. In a perfect world, the physician would always
be a person of exemplary moral integrity. Hippocrates would
have taken that as a given! In that world, there would be no need
for ethical rules at all. However, in reality, whereas moral rules
cannot be expected to pinch-hit for moral integrity, they do provide a point of reference for medical practitioners and the public
alike.

    Ideally, you the patient ought to be in partnership with the

Figure 1.1
A Model Ethical Decision-Making Process for Patients and Doctors

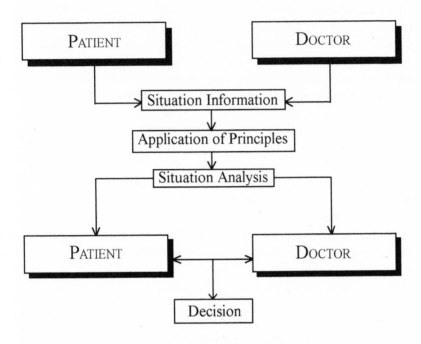

doctor who uses both ethical principles and situation ethics to come to the best decision in a given situation. Figure 1.1. shows the flow of information and the analysis that ought to take place in most situations in which an ethical dilemma occurs. Both the physician and the patient have equal, but different, roles to play. The physician is charged with the responsibility of providing the patient with understandable information about the medical aspects of the predicament, and the patient is charged with the responsibility of revealing all information pertinent to the situation to the physician. Together, they will look at the principles that govern the dilemmas and then, after independent analysis of the current situation, will make a decision together.

There is one more factor which must be considered in an overview of medical ethics as it is today – the fact that physicians face the conflict between the interests of the individual patient and those of society every day. The traditional approach of doing what is best for the patient (whatever that might be) will no longer suffice. Consider, for example, the case of the newly diagnosed epileptic patient who happens to be a pilot for a major airline. If the patient refuses to tell his employer about the problem and the doctor strictly maintains the patient's confidentiality, the lives of hundreds of unsuspecting people will be at risk each time that pilot takes to the skies. Is the physician's responsibility to one individual patient greater or less than his responsibility to society? This is a more common problem than many have previously considered. Often, the application of today's medical ethics has more of a social than an individual focus.

Obviously, there is more to your doctor's dilemmas than meets the eye. These are often complex problems that require well-developed decision-making abilities coupled with high personal moral integrity. The fact that doctors are only human leads us to believe that there may be a problem here.

How did your doctor learn to make ethical decisions? Next, we'll look at what your doctor *really* knows about ethics.

2

What Does a Doctor *Really* Know ... about Ethics?

Let's continue our visit with Dr Goode.

Dr Goode practises family medicine in a modern building that he moved into with his three partners five years ago. Attractively decorated, the office is also functional in design. His private office is his sanctuary. As you sit in front of his desk and look around you, you can see that Dr Goode is a very tidy person. Hung directly behind his head are two large, impressive-looking degrees, framed tastefully. If you understand any Latin at all, you will recognize that they are his undergraduate degree in science (his pre-med) and his medical degree. With its university insignia at the top and the red seal beside the official signatures at the bottom, the parchment tells you Dr Goode actually graduated from medical school and is the real thing. You never doubted it for a minute anyway.

But what does that degree really mean?

If you have never given much thought to those degrees hanging on the walls of your doctor's office, you are not alone. The very fact that this man or woman holds him or herself out as a physician is enough for most people to assume that he or she has the necessary education and training and will provide at least adequate medical care. What, then, is necessary education and training for a physician?

A medical degree implies two general things. First, your doctor has obtained enough basic arts and science credits at university to be admitted to a medical school. The basic requirements for admission to medical school are changing. Traditionally, they have included university courses in such subjects as biology, chemistry, physics, and often English, psychology, and electives chosen by the student. This would have been the experience of most doctors practising medicine today. But tomorrow's doctors may have a slightly different perspective. Recognizing that an all-science background doesn't necessarily make the best doctors, many medical schools are broadening their entrance requirements to recognize the contributions of social sciences and the arts.

The bottom line is, however, that a candidate for medical school has to have enough smarts to make it through a program that throws a great deal of information at students and in a very short time. Most students entering medical school have actually completed an undergraduate degree, but, at least in the past, having done so is not among the bare minimum requirements. Competition for entrance to medical school is keen, however, and the completion of a degree is often necessary for admission.

After these entrance requirements have been completed, a new medical student embarks upon four years (fewer in programs that run all year long) of medical training. The volume of material one must learn to complete the medical degree is enormous. Most of what medical students learn and are examined on prior to graduation, and subsequently prior to being granted a licence to practice, is the science of medicine. Where, then, does the *art* of medicine come in? How is your physician's ability to make compassionate, ethical decisions evaluated? Most medical schools rotate their students through so many situations and clinical tutors that it is difficult to make a valid measurement based on objective criteria.

For many years, people have believed that there must be something inherently 'ethical' about anyone who is a physician. As an editorial in *The Medical Post*, a newspaper for doctors, says: 'there has long been a comforting syllogism between the words "ethics" and "medicine." Patients and their families take reassurance from this implicit link and most doctors, I'm sure, do only "the right thing" for the people whose immediate and future existence is in their hands' (Pole 1989, 10).

The question remains: is this good enough for you? Is it good enough for you to believe that there is something inherently ethical about the practice of medicine, or have you come to the conclusion, and rightly so, that doctors are only human? They are not gods, and not saints; nor do they have a monopoly on the ability to make the right decision when dealing with thorny medical issues. What you need to know about them is how doctors perceive ethics, the problems they face every day, and what it is you can expect a doctor to have studied prior to hanging out a shingle.

ETHICS AND THE MEDICAL SCHOOLS

Since 1970, the ethical dilemmas posed by modern medical practice seem to be so great that some kind of formal education in ethics has become a common part of the curriculum in most North American medical schools. In 1976, an American Medical Association survey found that only 63 of the 113 medical schools in their study offered formal training in ethics theory. By the 1982–3 academic year, of 127 schools surveyed, all but one offered ethics, and 73 of the schools offered it as an elective. Giving future doctors a choice about whether or not to study ethics might seem odd. However, there is far from universal agreement on the value, if any, of formal ethics courses, and the courses themselves vary in content and approach. Indeed, there is a fundamental difference between teaching someone *about ethics* and teaching someone *to behave ethically.*

Another study, reported in 1985, examined 1,000 practising physicians who had graduated between 1974 and 1978 (Pellegrino and colleagues 1985). With close to a decade of practice behind them, the respondents were in a position to evaluate, at least to a degree, the extent to which ethics training had affected their abilities to make difficult decisions.

First, of 3,000 questionnaires that were mailed out, only 35 per cent, or about 1,050, were returned. Of those who did respond, only 30 per cent reported having received any formal training in ethics. In fact, the factors that seemed to have the most significant effect on their approaches to solving ethical dilemmas were personal values and beliefs, general clinical experience, role-model observation, family background, and interaction with peers. You may be surprised to know that formal course work in medical ethics and related topics rated lowest in their estimation of what affected their decisions most. Remember, though, few actually had any formal training in ethics. Clearly, then, who your physician is, where he or she comes from, and what makes him or her tick are very important – probably more so than any formal training in ethics.

In a related Canadian study of 300 physicians, 60 per cent of whom were practising family doctors, the researchers were interested in three aspects of ethical awareness (Balkos 1983). One of those aspects was the need for training in medical ethics. An overwhelming 81 per cent of those who took part in the study felt that they faced ethical problems in their daily practice, but the other 19 per cent said they had *no ethical problems at all.* You might wonder if that is, indeed, possible in medicine today. Thirty per cent of those who did recognize ethical dilemmas in their practices said that they would solve the problems on their own, and a further 43 per cent indicated that they would consult with a medical colleague. As far as codes of ethics and the ever-popular Hippocratic Oath are concerned, two-thirds of them had not taken the oath at all, and of those who had taken the oath at their graduations, two-thirds of them couldn't recall what it contained. As many as 68 per cent had never even read the Canadian Medical Association's Code of Ethics.

Both formal teaching of ethical theory and education in practical ethical decision making have peculiar places in the curricula of most medical schools. As we have noted already though, if your physician graduated before 1970, this discussion is academic, as courses in ethics probably did not have a place beside those in physiology, microbiology, pharmacology, and the like. In addition, the experience of medical school itself has been shown to have a rather unusual effect on attitudes of budding physicians towards medical ethics.

In one study, students were given an attitude questionnaire on their first day of medical school, and again near the end of their fourth year, prior to graduation (Tiberius and Cleave-Hogg 1984). The results were very interesting. The bright-eyed fledgling medical students in their first year indicated that they would be likely to look to an ethicist, or even the ethics literature, to help them to make ethical decisions in their future practice. After four years of the study of the science of medicine, though, the same students felt they would be less likely to need assistance in making moral decisions. An outsider might have expected just the opposite. One might have assumed that, as medical students were exposed to the myriad ethical dilemmas in the practice of modern medicine, they would look more positively on the possibility of advice from experts. That was not the case in this study.

A 1989 symposium on medical ethics in the medical school brought together medical school administrators and faculty for the specific purpose of discussing the ethics content of the curricula. Although all agreed that there was a need to teach ethics to future doctors, few agreed on what should be taught and how to teach it. In addition, some participants indicated that lack of both time and money was a barrier to the teaching of ethics. Perhaps more disturbing, though, was the citing of negative attitudes on the part of faculty and lack of information about the topic as barriers. It seemed clear that ethics education for future doctors had not been a priority for the majority of the medical educators represented at the conference (Lynch 1989).

The late Norman Cousins, a well-known author and educator, coined the phrase 'the barracuda syndrome,' to describe the psychology of the medical student today. With competition for admission and the ever-present need to make the grade, he says, 'students tend to know more about diseases than about the people in whom the diseases exist'; further, with the academic pressure of medical school, coupled with the sheer volume of the workload, 'these students are becoming drones rather than fully developed human beings ... they have time only to pursue the habits of grade-grabbing' (Cousins 1988, 79).

Although most of us would like to think that our own doctors did well academically, even in today's world of high-tech medicine we need to know that the physician has the capacity to care. Would you prefer a physician who made straight As, and in the process lost some measure of humanity, or a physician who did less well academically and cares who you are as a person? All of us have to decide individually what it is we are willing to settle for, but we can do that only if we understand the person beside the examining table, wearing the white coat and the stethoscope.

Several medical schools have experimented with ways for returning a modicum of humanity to the practice of medicine. Some of these experiments include attempting to add more intellectual stimulation to the curriculum and, as the Johns Hopkins University School of Medicine has done (for the class that began its studies in 1986), dropping the requirement for aspiring medical students to take the MCAT, the Medical College Admission Tests used by North American medical schools to screen applicants. Their decision was prompted by the belief that the preparation required for success on these tests discouraged applicants from taking courses in the humanities and led them, instead, to stick strictly to the pure sciences. From a medical school's point of view, this is a very daring decision, and the jury is still out on its value.

Before we can determine what ought to be taught to medical students about ethical decision making, it is necessary to make a distinction between the teaching of ethics and the teaching of ethical behaviour. If medical schools tell us, as consumers, that they are teaching ethical behaviour, there needs to be some evidence that the behaviour has been learned, just as we have a right to expect that a doctor who has been taught to remove an inflamed appendix can, in fact, remove that appendix successfully. However, the current situation is that ethical decision making is not effectively examined, if at all.

In real terms, even proven mastery of ethical theory is no reassurance. No matter how case-oriented and practicality-based an ethics curriculum might be on paper, there is no guarantee that the theory can be applied in practice by those who are charged with learning it. Indeed, all we, as consumers, can realistically expect is that the doctor in whose hands we may place our lives knows something about the theories that make up philosophical thought. How that individual makes that ethical decision – say, about who should get the only available organ for transplant – will be based on a set of personal moral values that were probably fixed, without critical thought, before his or her first day at medical school. When your values conflict with those of your doctor, a very real problem arises.

TAKING THE OATH ...

One of the expectations the average health care consumer has about the delivery of ethical health care is that the doctor (or nurse, or pharmacist, etc.) will follow some sort of a code of behaviour or will have taken an oath of some sort, and that failure to follow that code or adhere to that oath will result in disciplinary action. Such a perception presupposes a somewhat low level of moral development on the part of the health care provider. Nevertheless, most people seem to take some degree of comfort in believing that these codes and oaths will protect them. Let's look, then, at the Hippocratic Oath and some of these codes.

Generally considered to be the 'Father of Medicine,' Hippocrates was a Greek physician who lived during the latter part of the fifth century B.C. Many of his writings and those of his school have survived, the most famous of which is the Hippocratic Oath, which originated with his teachings and has come to be known as the ethical guide of the medical profession.

The Hippocratic Oath, which is taken in a modified form by many, but by no means all, graduating doctors, has a preamble which begins: 'I swear by Apollo, the Physician, by Aesculapius, by Hygeia, by Panacea, by all the gods and goddesses, to keep, according to my ability and judgement, the following Oath.' This preamble is the very heart of the problem with the oath. The phrase 'according to my ability and judgement' implies that there is nothing absolute about the duties that follow, and thus provides an 'out.' A physician whose level of competence does not allow him or her to 'prescribe regimen for the good of my patients ... and never do anyone harm' cannot reasonably be expected to do so. The issue thus becomes one of medical ability.

Codes of medical ethics have been described as guidelines for exemplary physician behaviour and that definition is probably the closest to the truth of any attempts to define them. Codes of ethics have been developed by professional associations of physicians to control the relationships of doctors with other doctors, and the relationships of doctors with patients. These codes, however, can hardly be viewed as articulations of major philosophical principles.

The American Medical Association's original code mentioned the patient in the first paragraph, but was primarily concerned about the relationship of physicians with each other. Emphasis on the patient has increased since the inception of the code, but if practising physicians can't remember what the code says anyway, it can hardly be held out as the basis for their ethical decision making.

The original Code of Ethics of the Canadian Medical Association was adopted at the first annual meeting of the association, held in September 1868. In the minutes of that meeting, the Code of Medical Ethics, which followed fairly closely the AMA code, consisted of sections relating to:

1. The duties of physicians to their patients and of the *obligations of patients to their physicians*;
2. The duties of physicians to each other and to the profession at large;
3. The duties of the profession to the public and of the *obligations of the public to the profession*. (emphasis added)

The major differences between the original and the current codes are that the original code paid more attention to compassion and caring, obligations of the patient to the physician, delineation of duties of the patient, and etiquette. The current code (1990 edition) also has three sections:

1. Responsibilities to the patient;
2. Responsibilities to the profession;
3. Responsibilities to society.

While the provisions of the codes of ethics for physicians put forward a commendable list of dos and don'ts for the conduct of a practice, there are two very glaring problems with them: first, as we have said, many doctors – perhaps more than we know – are wholly unaware of what their code has to say; and, second, the codes offer few guidelines for the practical decision making required of physicians on a daily basis.

As a self-regulating group, the medical profession has, in its codes of ethics, a powerful public relations tool. Like society in general, physicians have diverse points of view, and from the perspective of medical politics, codes are of necessity vague in their language. This lack of clarity allows for differences of opinion to exist within the same moral framework. As useful as this may be for the ethics committees of professional medical associations, it is often not very comforting to the patient. On the other hand, the fact that this assortment of opinions exists gives the patient the opportunity to seek out and find a doctor who shares his or her perspectives.

Let's look at a few of the specific provisions of North American medical codes of ethics and determine what questions they raise, as opposed to what answers they give.

- 'An ethical physician shall, except in an emergency, have the right to refuse to accept a patient' (Canadian code); 'A physician may choose whom he will serve. In an emergency, however, he should render service to the best of his ability' (American code).

  Doesn't that mean that a physician has no obligation to treat a patient with AIDS, to provide an abortion or even referral for one, to treat a patient of a different racial extraction, etc.?
- 'An ethical physician will keep in confidence information derived from a patient or from a colleague regarding a patient, and divulge it only with the permission of the patient except when otherwise required by law' and 'An ethical physician will

strive to improve standards of medical services in the community; will accept a share of the profession's responsibility to society in matters relating to the health and safety of the public ...' (Canadian code).

Don't these two provisions come into conflict when a patient's condition can potentially have harmful effects on larger numbers of people, as in the case of a patient with AIDS or a commercial airline pilot prone to epileptic seizures?

The code of the American Medical Association deals with this issue by stating: 'A physician may not reveal the confidences entrusted to him ... unless he is required to do so by law *or unless it becomes necessary in order to protect the welfare of the individual or the community* [emphasis added].' In both codes, the provisions for confidentiality place a doctor in a very difficult position.

As you can see, some of the provisions of the codes do little to simplify the ethical decision-making process and often muddy the waters. It seems clear that a doctor's knowledge of a Code of Ethics is no guarantee of an ability to make morally correct, or at least defensible, decisions. We might listen to the former director of Ethics and Legal Affairs for the Canadian Medical Association, who has said of codes of ethics, they 'pose a threat because they are substitutes for ethical reasoning' (Kluge 1992, 1234).

THE DOCTOR, THE PERSON

What is likely to have the most significant impact on an individual doctor's approach to ethical dilemmas is the personal value system of that person – those values and attitudes that have developed over the life of the doctor and wend their way into the thought processes of each of us. Among the factors that affect an individual's attitudes and personal values are:

1. cultural background
2. educational experiences and interests
3. family structure and dynamics

4. religious upbringing
5. social class, both past and present
6. race
7. personal characteristics

It is the unique combination of these factors that makes each human being different from the next. Although they may share some things, even children brought up in the same household perceive experiences in different ways, and the individual's personality will colour the perceptions, leading to the development of different values. These are the characteristics that each fledgling medical student brings to the experience of medical school, and many of these are pretty well carved in stone at that time. Some attitudes are so entrenched that nothing that the medical school can offer will change those. In fact, some medical educators believe that morality is a matter of predispositions.

Another factor that must be considered is the level of moral development of an individual physician. Just as we develop social skills and thinking skills throughout our lives, we also develop moral skills that guide our behaviour.

Psychologist Lawrence Kohlberg put forward a widely used theory to explain why people make moral decisions the way they do. He believes that moral development encompasses an expansion of one's concerns to an ever-widening range of people and interests. For example, at a very young age a child learns that it is wrong to steal and is able to resist doing so not because he or she sees anything inherently wrong with stealing, or that it will have negative effects on other people, but because he or she has learned from experience that those who steal are punished. Kohlberg would say that this indicates a very rudimentary level of moral reasoning, a stage we all go through and one that, unfortunately, many people never progress beyond.

At a higher level of moral reasoning, an individual will make a decision either to satisfy a need to be judged a good person by others or to fulfil duties that have been agreed upon to keep the system running. A physician who relies on a series of rules to govern ethical decisions could be thought of as being at this level, maintaining the status quo.

At the highest stages of moral development, an individual is able to see the bigger picture, to apply universal moral principles *for the good of society.* We would all like to think that our doctors function at this high level of moral development but, sadly, that is probably not so. In fact, not many people do function at this level on a regular basis. We all regress to the level of the young child who makes the right decision simply because of a need to avoid being punished. How many people stay within the speed limit when driving on the highway because they recognize the potential danger to others of high speed? Could the motive for staying within the speed limit often be the desire to avoid being caught? The proliferation of radar-detection devices in cars today seems to supply the answer.

Although this way of thinking about a human being's moral development helps us to understand how ethical decisions might be made, it doesn't tell the whole story. Another consideration is the extent to which a person can be aware that he or she is, indeed, facing a question of ethics. Other concerns include how the individual judges what is right, and whether the person has the personal strength of convictions to see that his or her beliefs are followed through on (Rest 1986).

Researchers have looked at the moral development of medical students. In one study, researchers tested a group of medical students at the beginning of their first year and again at the end of their last year to find out their moral-reasoning scores. The results indicated that the students failed to show even the normally expected increase in moral-reasoning scores for people who continue their formal education. Medical school had somehow interfered with their moral-reasoning ability instead of helping it to develop (Self and colleagues 1993). The same group of researchers looked at the effects of incorporating a formal medical ethics course into the medical curriculum. This study found that students who received a formal course in medical ethics actually improved their scores on a moral-reasoning test (Self and colleagues 1992). These researchers concluded that it is possible to develop young people's moral reasoning in medical school.

What does all this mean in determining what your own doctor really knows about ethics? First and foremost, it means that graduation from a recognized medical school does not guarantee ethical competence, but that more recent graduates are likely to have been exposed to formal ethics education. Those who did not receive this training may be able to offset this lack by their experience since graduation. Second, what makes your doctor tick as a person may be more important in the long run than the number of medical ethics courses he or she has taken. Third, it is not enough for a physician to have good intentions in making decisions; those decisions must be based on competence in both the medical/scientific component of the practice of medicine and the philosophical/compassionate component of the art of medicine.

In summary, your physician needs to have the following:

1. the ability to know when an ethical problem exists
2. the ability to analyse conflicting rights and obligations
3. a workable framework for decision making
4. a commitment to include the patient in that decision-making process
5. an ability to identify situations in which his or her personal values conflict with a patient's

Identifying these characteristics here is the easy part. Finding out how your own doctor measures up is much harder.

WHAT YOU CAN DO

• Start by asking your doctor (and especially any new doctor you might consult) a few simple questions, such as: How often do you confront ethical problems in your everyday practice? If he or she tells you that it never happens, you need to be concerned that the little things are getting by unnoticed.
• Read the newspapers, watch the television newscasts, or lis-

ten to the radio news. Read the health-related magazines in your doctor's waiting-room. Talk to your doctor about issues that you read, see, or hear about. As the doctor is taking your blood pressure or doing your pap smear, you might start the conversation about any number of issues that make their way into the media, ranging from organ donation to euthanasia. Listen for your doctor's degree of understanding and ability to impart this to you.

- Ask your doctor what he or she might do in situations similar to those receiving media coverage. Does the answer seem to be well thought out? Is the doctor interested in discussing these issues at all?
- Listen closely for value judgments. Which position on the issue does your doctor think is right or wrong? Is he or she open-minded or opinionated? If the latter, do those opinions reflect your own point of view?
- Always be observant when you are visiting your doctor. You may hear your doctor talking about ethics-related issues without your having to mention them.

The bottom line is that you need to be well informed and you have to speak up when you want an answer. If you are curious about what is being taught today in a medical school about a particular topic, ask your doctor, or call the closest medical school. With today's concerns about public image, even medical schools cannot afford to turn a deaf ear to curious consumers.

3

Doctor and Patient:
A Unique Relationship

When Dr Goode returned to his private office after his lunch meeting, he found that his receptionist, as usual, had placed on his desk a stack of mail as well as a stack of charts. He sighed as he noted, yet again, that a large proportion of his mail seemed to be that unsolicited variety that would fill his wastebasket. Nevertheless, he would get to it later this afternoon. He sat back and began to refresh his memory with the charts of the patients he was about to see.

The first patient was there for a well-baby visit. He had delivered this baby only two weeks earlier, and now the mother was bringing him, a healthy boy, in for the standard check-up.

The second patient would be a bit more out of the ordinary. Michelle Smith was a twenty-one-year-old, senior university student. Two months ago she had arrived in his office complaining of headaches. After carrying out a thorough physical examination and taking some blood samples to rule out some possibilities that Dr Goode thought unlikely anyway, he had spent some time talking with her. She had just broken up with her fiancé and was facing the uncertainty of an application to graduate school, and her father had died during the semester. This information, coupled with her description of the band-like, constricting nature of the headaches themselves, had led Dr Goode to the diagnosis of tension headaches. As he now recalled, Ms Smith did not agree. She had insisted upon seeing a specialist for a second opinion.

It had been clear to Dr Goode that, despite his having been her family physician for many years, she did not trust his judgment. He suspected that she did not like the idea of not being able to cope with the events in her life and had convinced herself that she had some underlying neurological problem.

Dr Goode had found himself in a dilemma that day. Thirty years ago the patient would not have asked for a second opinion, and although Dr Goode usually welcomed a patient's involvement in his or her own medical care, he had not felt that Ms Smith's condition warranted it. In fact, he had wondered if it would even be ethical to comply with her request, knowing as he did about the waiting-list for neurologists in town. He also knew, however, that he was bound to help his patient even though others might be in greater need. So, he had made the appointment.

Ms Smith had seen the neurologist three weeks ago, and the specialist's letter about the visit had arrived yesterday. According to the consultant, Ms Smith not only had insisted that her problem was neurological, but had made such a fuss about having a CAT scan that he had squeezed her in ahead of some of his other patients. Just as he had predicted, the results of the CAT scan were normal, as were all the other findings. His diagnosis: tension headaches. Now she was coming back to Dr Goode, complaining of headaches yet again.

When Ms Smith walked into Dr Goode's office, she looked healthy and relaxed. But she was a very unhappy lady. She told Dr Goode that she thought the neurologist was a quack, and she wanted an MRI – she knew they had a new machine at the hospital – and another opinion.

Dr Goode's first reaction was to tell her that she had received all that the high-tech, modern medical diagnostic arsenal had to offer her and then to discuss with her how they might go about treating the tension headaches. But a small part of him said: What if I'm wrong? What if the consultant and I are both wrong? But how long can we continue to second-guess ourselves?

What *should* Dr Goode do? What would you, as a patient, expect of him in a similar situation? After all, he is the one who spent all those years studying to be a doctor. After all, he is the one in whom you have placed a certain amount of trust and with whom you have built a relationship over a period of time. It is the doctor's responsibility to keep you safe and well. Or is it? Have you placed trust in this doctor or not? One surgeon put it this way: 'Today, doctors are supposed to be perfect even if patients are not. They are expected to communicate well, even with patients who are vengeful and justify their attitude with the belief that doctors have huge incomes ... It is time to educate the public, to inform people that they may contribute to their own illness' (Devroede 1991, 56). Clearly, doctors feel the change in patients' attitudes, and these attitudes often make it difficult for doctors to do what they truly believe is best for the patient. The relationship is certainly not what it used to be.

Recent changes in the field of medicine, ranging from high-technology advances to the growth of consumerism, to fear of litigation, to increased media interest in reporting apparent ethical transgressions of doctors, have conspired to change the way that patients relate to physicians. And, although not all of these changes have been detrimental, they have changed that sacred, fundamental relationship that has always been the corner-stone of medical treatment. In a 1989 *Time* magazine article about doctors, titled aptly enough 'Sick and Tired,' the author, Nancy Gibbs (1989), put it this way: 'Never have doctors been able to do so much for their patients, and rarely have patients seemed so ungrateful.'

Let's look, first, at the differences between the professional relationship that you would have with a health-care worker and the personal one you might have with a friend. Some people believe that a professional relationship is one that, by definition, is distant, impersonal, and rather cold, but nevertheless competent. This probably does not come close to the description that most of us would like to apply to our relationships with our personal physicians. On the other hand, a personal relationship might be characterized by physical and emotional closeness, both of which could be seen to hinder a doctor's objectivity in his or her treatment of a patient. Ideally, then, how should your doctor relate to you?

A doctor should be able to blend those professional qualities that are held in such high esteem by colleagues, such as knowledge, technical ability, efficiency, objectivity, and competence, with human qualities, such as warmth, understanding, and compassion. It is these human qualities in the competent physician that make him or her stand out from all the others.

There are times, however, when the good doctor should work to create a distance between him or herself and the patient in an attempt to do what is best for the patient. Some of those times are:

1. when a patient is lonely. Doctors who do not put some distance between themselves and the lonely patient run the risk of becoming that person's constant companion. This is not healthy for the doctor, the patient, or the doctor's relationship with other patients.
2. when a doctor feels pity for the patient. In these situations, the doctor runs the risk of becoming so emotionally involved that objectivity in treatment is totally lost.
3. when a doctor overidentifies with a patient. This is a particular problem when a doctor has had an experience that is very similar to the patient's. Patients often feel that a doctor who has actually experienced a particular situation is likely better able to handle it in the patient. This is not necessarily so. In fact, it is more likely to cloud the doctor's objectivity.
4. when the patient is a social acquaintance or a family member. Some doctors find it almost impossible to be objective and professional when dealing with people who are well known to them outside the office. A good doctor will usually refuse to treat family members and will be very cautious about treating friends. There are only a very few legitimate situations in which doctors must treat family members or close friends, including the one-doctor small town and emergencies. Otherwise, this should not occur.

Over the years, a great deal of thought has been given to the types of relationships that patients have had with their doctors, and typically these have changed over time. Before we discuss these relationships, though, we should examine several characteristics that are common to this unique bond. The first characteristic is that, regardless of how you relate to your individual physician, the relationship is one-to-one. Whether or not your doctor treats other members of your family, your relationship with him or her is singular.

The second thing that these relationships have in common is that the patient asks for it. Except in very specific circumstances, such as where the patient is unconscious, he or she presents him or herself for consultation with the physician. The doctor then sets up the specifics of when and where the relationship will be carried through. The result is that the physician takes on the dominant role, and the patient a more or less passive, or at least secondary, one. How you view this configuration of roles depends upon who you are, where you come from, and what experiences you have had. There are cultural as well as regional differences in what the consumer expects of his or her doctor, and your attitude will reflect all of these unique characteristics.

Traditionally, communication within the doctor–patient relationship has been either one-way (coming from the doctor to the patient) or two-way (doctor and patient each give information/feedback to the other). Using this knowledge, and the fact that many attempts have been made in the medical literature to describe these relationships for physicians, we present to you our models of the doctor–patient relationship. Perhaps you will see your relationship with your doctor among them.

THE PARENT–CHILD RELATIONSHIP

In simpler times, the majority of doctor–patient relationships were based on the parent–child model. The doctor believed he or she knew best, and the patient agreed. Conflicts were few, but one has to wonder if the best care was forthcoming in such a lopsided setting. Even if the doctor generally had the best interests of the patient at heart and in mind, the lack of patient input made the medical decision something that was done *to* the patient instead of *with* him or her. Even today, some physicians bemoan the fact that this is no longer the universally accepted relationship.

THE SALESPERSON–CUSTOMER RELATIONSHIP

The objective in this model is for the customer (the patient) to get what he or she thinks is needed. The salesperson (the doctor) sells what he or she needs to sell. Obviously, a great deal of persuasive communication is sometimes required for this model to work to the advantage of the salesperson, but it is not always difficult to convince the customer of what he or she ought to be buying and that it is the right thing to do. Medical and health problems are so personal and can be so threatening that the patient will often be more than willing to buy what the doctor has to sell.

THE TEAM

In this model, both parties agree upon the goal of the care and respect each other's ability to achieve that goal. There is an implied contract, and the decision making is shared. For this relationship to work, however, each party (doctor and patient) has to hold up his or her end honestly. The onus is not solely on the doctor, but is shared by the patient. There are no stars here, only partners in care.

TREATING THE PATIENT/TREATING THE DISEASE

Clearly, the pendulum is swinging. On one side is the view that the sickness must be treated (the traditional medical view). On the other side is the view that the patient as a person must be treated (the holistic view). Each of these views, in the extreme, has an effect on the doctor–patient relationship. When only the disease is considered, to the exclusion of the patient as a person, the patient loses rights. And, although one might think that the holistic approach that views the whole person in concert with the environment is the way to approach medical decision making, don't forget that, to a very large extent, the traditional medical approach brought us to our current understanding of disease processes in the body.

What effect is this new relationship having? Neither all patients nor all doctors like the idea that the physician no longer tells the unquestioning patient what to do. Some patients have difficulty dealing with the expectation that they will be partners in care, and some physicians still expect patients to take every one of their words at face value. Obviously, a patient who wants to have a say in his or her care will be in conflict with a traditionally paternalistic doctor.

The baby-boom generation – the population swell between 1947 and 1966 – has had an enormous impact on this changing relationship. While their parents might have shown deference for doctors, the boomers are right in there, swinging their axes at the bases of the pedestals, attempting to topple the doctors, who are hanging on for dear life. An official with the polling organization Environics has been quoted as saying, 'Baby boomers are less likely to be deferential to people whose professional credentials suggest they should be deferred to' (Ubelacker 1993, B2). These controllers of the trends are looking more to self-help. As a result, even professional associations of medical practitioners seem to have decided that there is merit in this new interest that patients have been showing in taking control of their own health decisions. For example, some professional medical associations have begun publishing self-help books on everything from prescription drugs to baby and mother care.

Most people agree that it is beneficial for the patient to have a greater role in decision making. In today's consumer environment, it seems that physicians who refuse to allow this participation should be disciplined. Indeed, the requirement that doctors need to have the 'informed' consent of patients to perform procedures moves in this direction.

MODERN THREATS

Six modern factors are currently threatening or at least affecting the sanctity of your relationship with your doctor. In fact, these factors are often the cause of the dilemmas with which your doctor must deal. They are:

1. patients' expectations and consumerism;
2. media reporting;
3. doctors' fear of litigation;
4. advances in medical technology;
5. doctors' fear of losing patients;
6. doctors' 'job actions' or strikes.

Patients' expectations of modern medical technology have had a major impact on the new doctor–patient relationship. We may be healthier today than we have ever been in history, but we are also more apprehensive about our health, and this affects how we relate to our health care providers. One of the things that has contributed to this nervousness is the news media. For a large portion of the North American population, the news media, both print and broadcast, are the major source of information about health-related matters. While the mass media can be a powerful tool in informing the public about medical issues, not all of what is reported in the press is information that is useful for everyone. It's important to keep in mind that, when the press reports a 'medical breakthrough,' the label is theirs and is not necessarily one that the medical community would apply. On the other hand, it can only benefit your care to discuss with your physician what you read, see, or hear about in the media.

It is becoming well known in medical circles that most medical malpractice suits launched by patients are a result of poor communication with their physicians and that few of them are initiated as a result of lapses in medical judgment. Clearly, a physician who takes the time to explain things to patients is more likely to be perceived as doing the right thing. Both patients and doctors need to be aware of how important this communication is.

The seemingly large number of medical malpractice suits that has become a reality in recent years is in itself having an impact on how our physicians relate to us. Consider again Dr Goode's dilemma at the beginning of this chapter. If he felt little threat of being sued, he might be more inclined to make what he clearly considers the best decision both for this patient and for the others who truly are in need of more specialized help. Whereas, in his best judgment Ms Smith does not need to see yet another specialist, knowing that he might be sued, Dr Goode is more likely to make the referral. Threat of litigation seems like a poor basis on which to make a medical decision.

Advances in medical technology have had a number of effects on the doctor–patient relationship. First, the rapidly growing knowledge base of medicine means that each physician has to scurry just to keep up with what's new. Doctors need continually to ask themselves if they are truly up-to-date. Second, this move to reliance on high-tech medicine, in part as a response to patient demand and in part because those who make the advances promote their use, has forced an emotional wedge between the patient and the doctor. Dependence upon the science rather than the art of medicine has changed the complexion of that relationship. Physicians who rely on technology and the so-called quick fix for everything from a hangnail to heart disease have distanced themselves from what they need more than anything else – patients.

Another factor that affects the modern doctor–patient relationship is the threat of increasing competition and the consequent fear some doctors have of losing patients. As more and more doctors graduate from medical school and set up practices, parts of North America, especially urban areas, are becoming oversupplied with doctors. The result has been a mind-set that often leads doctors to see patients in terms of how much income they represent. There is no question that this perception can affect the quality of the care, including the amount of time a doctor gives to an individual patient's complaint. On the plus side, competition has made it crucial for doctors to be able not only to attract patients but also to maintain them, and the tactics they may use in pursuing this goal, ranging from issuing patient newsletters to offering specialized services in their offices, can only serve to improve the overall delivery of care.

The expanding roles of other health care professionals are also contributing to doctors' fear of losing patients. Nurses, physiotherapists, nutritionists, health educators, pharmacists, and so on have increased their profiles over the past decade, and are looking for their own areas of authority. Some doctors see this as an infringement on their traditional medical role, and the result has been some hostile feelings between the professions. A doctor who confidently asks for the opinions and input of other professionals is likely to be the doctor who is the most sure of him or herself and the least susceptible to the fear of losing patients.

One last modern contrivance that has insinuated itself into the relationship between doctor and patient is the 'job action' or strike. The trade-union approach to accomplishing specific objectives has filtered into even the sacred pact that a doctor has to 'consider first the well-being of the patient.' Some of the rationales doctors have given for going on strike have included bringing pressure to bear on governments for a variety of reasons, lowering malpractice insurance premiums, decreasing the number of hours worked, and improving the efficiency of medical assistance.

The bottom line is that these walk-outs, slow-downs, and general obstructions to medical care have resulted, not in positive public opinion in support of doctors and their quests, but in a general questioning of medical commitment. Despite this perception, there is another, very real side to this story – namely, that doctors may truly have the best interests of the patients at heart when deciding to take such action. Their concerns for the long term may override their belief in the need to provide uninterrupted care in the short term.

So you can see that, each time you walk into your doctor's

office, numerous factors play a part in the outcome of that encounter. The extent to which you allow these factors to affect your own personal relationship with your doctor depends on how seriously you have evaluated your physician's philosophy of patient care.

WHAT YOU CAN DO

As in any relationship between two people, neither one can have complete control over the outcome of any encounter. Interaction between human beings simply has too many unpredictable aspects. There are, however, some measures that you can take to increase the likelihood that you will have the type of relationship that you want and to play an equal part in decision making.

• Be forthright with your doctor about how you would like to be addressed. If you feel more comfortable being called 'Mrs Smith' than 'Debbie,' tell your doctor.
• Avoid socializing with your doctor. If you end up in the same social circle, it might be a good idea to find another doctor.
• Avoid discussing your medical problems with family members who happen to be doctors. Such discussions put both of you in an awkward situation.
• When you decide that you need a second opinion (which is your right), explain your desire without implying that you distrust your primary-care physician.
• Try to keep an open mind about what you read in the newspapers about the ethical transgressions of doctors. Each doctor is an individual and should be judged on his or her own merits.
• If you feel uncomfortable with how your doctor is treating you, find another doctor.

4
Keeping Secrets

Imagine yourself visiting your doctor's office to discuss your pap smear, your prostate, your nervous condition, your back injury, your bed-wetting child, or any other health concern that you might have. Your belief in your doctor's absolute commitment to keeping your secrets is one of the main reasons that you will feel, if not completely at ease, at least satisfied that your confidence will be kept. This has been true since there have been physicians. Consider what you would do if you thought that your doctor would be likely to walk through the office door and discuss your medical problems with his or her grocer, hair stylist, social acquaintances, or even his or her spouse. Would this change your relationship?

While most of us feel relatively comfortable that such betrayals of confidence are not likely to occur very often, we sometimes forget that there are many instances in modern health care in which the trust we accord our doctors may in fact be misplaced. Let us return to Dr Goode's office, this time seeing it as many of his patients might.

Mr Jones is thirty-five years old and has been married for five years. On a recent business trip, he had a brief sexual encounter with someone other than his wife for the first time since his wedding, and he now fears that he may have contracted a sexually transmitted disease. He visited Dr Goode a week ago for tests and a check-up, and now he is returning for the results. He is seated nervously in the waiting-room, trying to read a business magazine, but he is distracted by both his own thoughts and the receptionist's loud telephone conversation. 'What is the nature of your complaint today, Mrs White?' she was saying. She began using the keyboard in front of her to input information into the computer. 'You've run out of Valium? You know Dr Goode won't refill that prescription without an office visit ... I know you've been on it for some time, but he just won't do it ... He can see you tomorrow at three.'

At that point a white-coated woman arrived and dumped a sheaf of papers on the ledge of the reception desk.

'Mr Jones?' the receptionist called. 'Could I see you for a minute?'

He arose from his seat and walked over to the desk.

'Mr Jones, I have your record in front of me. It seems that we don't have an updated insurance number for you.'

Mr Jones began digging in his pocket, knocking several papers on the floor in the process. As he picked them up, he noticed that they were laboratory result sheets. Straightening himself up, he glanced at the computer screen and could see his name and a glimpse of his record that said, 'Diagnosis: Possible STD.' He couldn't see much else. He handed her his card and returned to his seat.

Another patient arrived at the desk to announce herself and began a friendly conversation with the receptionist. He realized that his record was probably still displayed on the computer screen. He began squirming in his seat.

Finally, it was his turn. After an eternal week of worrying, he was relieved to find that he was completely healthy. He left the office as quickly as he could, vowing never to get himself in such a predicament again. He got onto the elevator with two of the doctors' office employees and sighed with relief.

'Did you hear that Mrs MacDonald complaining?' one said to the other. 'If she'd stick to the diet and lose some weight, maybe she could get around better.'

'Oh, she's a lost cause,' her companion said. 'She had stomach stapling last year, for all the good it's done.' They both snickered.

Mr Jones fled the elevator to his waiting car.

I will not divulge anything that, in connection with my profession or otherwise, I may see or hear of the lives of men which should not be revealed, on the belief that all such things should be kept secret.
– The Oath of Hippocrates

For centuries, doctors and other health professionals have been advised, or rather warned, that patient information is strictly confidential. Modern times, however, have begun to dent that absolute value rather nastily. The scene in Dr Goode's office may seem a bit exaggerated, and it is likely that you will not see as many transgressions in one place, but each of these little problems happens every day. Before we examine the factors that are eroding this absolute value in modern medicine, we need to discuss what the concept of keeping secrets in medical practice means now, and has meant through the ages.

WHAT DOES CONFIDENTIALITY REALLY MEAN?

A patient's ability to feel comfortable that the intimate details of his or her life, told to a medical practitioner in confidence, will remain just that way is the corner-stone of the doctor–patient relationship. It has been that way for centuries. The trust that a patient has in the relationship is a fundamental part of the therapeutic connection.

While this notion seems simple and straightforward, modern medicine has considerable difficulty dealing with such absolutes, and the concept of maintaining a patient's confidence has become diluted in today's world of health care.

The International Code of Medical Ethics (1983) says that 'a doctor owes to his patient absolute secrecy on all which has been confided in him or which he knows because of confidences confided in him.' This seems fairly clear, but now consider the American Medical Association's Principles of Medical Ethics (1980), which says that a physician 'shall safeguard patient confidences within the constraints of the law,' and the Canadian

Medical Association's Code of Ethics (1990), which adds the caveat 'except when otherwise required by law.' At the time of this writing, the CMA's code is being reviewed to consider social responsibility to an even greater extent. It seems, then, that the 'absolute' of confidentiality is in fact conditional, and that several intervening variables come between the doctor and the patient. A patient can no longer expect unequivocally that his or her confidence will be kept in the context of a relationship with a personal physician. Whenever there is a question of whether the confidence of the patient might harm either the patient or others, doctors and other health professionals face a dilemma to which there is no easy answer and into which the patient has little, if any, input.

The problems that modern medicine has in keeping patients' secrets can be summed up in several questions:

- Is all information about a patient considered to be confidential, or only some of it?
- To whom is access to this information restricted?
- If a doctor tells a patient's secret to another doctor or health professional, under what circumstances has he or she broken that confidence?
- What are the limits of the individual patient's right to privacy?

While you might think that today's sophisticated system of health care would have answers for you, the patient, to these questions, the fact is that these issues are thorny still. The problem is further confounded by every new advance in medical treatment and technology. Each step forward is a step back in terms of resolving the quandary about keeping secrets.

WHAT IS ERODING OUR PRIVACY?

It would be easier for both doctor and patient if the edict that Hippocrates made about keeping patients' secrets could be followed at all times. There would be few dilemmas. In the twentieth century, however, doing so is not that easy or straightforward. One writer has put it this way: 'old-fashioned medical confidentiality has become a notion quaint as the house call – gradually eroded by court decisions and a victim of industrialization of medicine' (Norton 1989). Several factors have contributed to this erosion that both doctors and patients today face in their search for a confidential encounter. These include the increasing use of computers in medical care; legal requirements for reporting; occupational medicine; insurance company requirements; the need to generate research data; the proliferation of allied health professions; and an overriding public interest. We'll examine each one in more detail.

Computers
Computers have infiltrated many aspects of our everyday lives. Few businesses, even homes, today are without computers. Hospitals and doctors' offices are no different. Computers and electronic data are here in a big way, and they are arguably the most worrisome of the modern advances that threaten our privacy in many areas of life, including health care. The problems that computers pose for the protection of privacy in medical care have yet to be addressed satisfactorily by our doctors.

There is a story of a young University of Michigan student who was injured while cross-country skiing in a campus park. A native of Detroit, he had his computerized medical records sent to the hospital in Ann Arbor, where they discovered that he'd had his gall bladder removed at age two, among other unusual problems for such a young man. When all was sorted out, it became clear that the medical histories of both his grandfather and his uncle, all of whom shared the same name, had been lumped together by the computer (Norton 1989). While this error was easily corrected at the time, consider what might have happened had these data become a permanent part of a medical-history database at an insurance company.

One Oklahoma-based clearing-house stores and processes 1.5 million medical insurance claims monthly and provides health trend information for employers gleaned from these records of

6.3 million employees (Goldberg 1992). Considering the number of computer hackers who are able to get into the databases of banks, universities, and big businesses, we would be foolish to think that these computer networks are safe.

Even simple things like the degree to which the computer screen with a medical record on it can be seen by passers-by is of concern. Computer operators should be ensuring that the screen cannot be seen by anyone who isn't directly involved in your care, and that the screen is cleared after consultation with the record.

Computerization is also an important trend in hospital record-keeping. It has eased considerably the paper trails left behind by patients with long medical charts. These trails, paper-less though they may be today, are still there and are readily accessible to dozens of people, legitimately.

Legal Requirements for Reporting
Another significant erosion factor in patient confidentiality is legitimized by its mention in codes of ethics: namely, the need for legal reporting of certain conditions. For years physicians have been required by law to report certain medical conditions that may be deemed to be hazardous to the health of others. The most widely known of these has been sexually transmitted diseases. The reason for this reporting requirement was so that the wheels of the public-health process could be put into motion to trace the patient's sexual contacts, arranging for their treatment and preventing their unknowingly infecting others. This legal requirement has been very high profile in recent years as HIV (the virus that causes AIDS) carriers and their supporters have baulked at the idea of being identified to health officials. Their concerns are less about the health aspects of the problem, than the social problems created by public identification of people who carry the virus.

In a high-profile Canadian case, two physicians were ordered by the court to pay $290,000 (Cdn) each in damages to the family of a victim who died as a result of a motor-vehicle accident involving an epileptic driver. In their particular jurisdiction, physicians are required by law to report anyone who has a condition that might make it dangerous for him or her to operate a motor vehicle. In this case, the doctors failed to do so. Other reportable conditions in many jurisdictions also include the suspicion of physical or sexual abuse of children. In these cases, even the suspicion must be reported, and some laws extend to anyone, not just a doctor who suspects that a child is being abused.

Occupational Medicine
Occupational medicine is one of the newer factors that threatens the privacy of our medical information. Many of today's employers seem to think that they have a right to know about every employee's medical history. In fact, some even call their employees' private physicians directly in an attempt to gain information about the legitimacy of complaints resulting in sick time, the employees' claims for the need for a light workload, or anything else that might relate to the work situation. It certainly is not their right. Your medical record is not open to your employer unless you have expressly indicated in writing that it is, and your doctor knows that.

Insurance Company Requirements
Insurance company requirements can also be viewed as an eroder of doctor–patient confidentiality. While it is necessary for insurance companies to obtain medical information about applicants and claimants, medical practitioners do not have the right to give out information without seeing the actual permission form signed by the patient. On the other hand, a doctor does not have the right to withhold pertinent information about the patient in a misguided attempt to protect the patient from high insurance fees. If such action is discovered, both the doctor and the patient will be liable, and the insurance claim may not be paid.

The Need to Generate Research Data
The need to generate research data is one of the privacy problems that patients rarely know about. This is of particular con-

cern in large teaching hospitals affiliated with university medical schools when a medical researcher decides to do a retrospective study of patients who have suffered from a particular condition over a period of, say, ten years. The records of all the identified patients are pulled, and research assistants comb the charts, looking for particular pieces of information. Even though individual patients will never be identifiable, the issue of permission to have unknown persons who are not involved in your care be given access to your charts often never surfaces.

Even medical journals receive papers that have been written about studies of questionable ethical value. In a 1992 editorial in the *Canadian Medical Association Journal*, the editor relates two examples (Squires 1992). The first was the report of a study during which the researchers asked the doctors in a particular town to give them the names of patients who suffered from the condition they wished to study. The doctors did this, and the researchers wrote to the patients. It was clear that these patients had not given their doctors permission to divulge their names in the first place. In the second study, the researchers went directly to the hospital charts to find people who fit into their studies; then, they approached these patients' doctors to ask permission to contact the patients. The appropriate sequence would have been to ask doctors to identify suitable patients, secure their permission, and then relate their individual responses to the researchers. The frightening thing for you, the patient, should be the fact that many medical practitioners saw nothing at all wrong with either approach.

The Proliferation of Allied Health Professionals
The proliferation of allied health professionals is another problem in patient confidentiality. Do you remember the old game we used to play as children? It started with a secret whispered in the ear of one person. As the secret was told and retold around a circle, it was embellished to the point that it bore little resemblance to the original version. When numerous health professionals are involved in an individual's medical care, a similar phenomenon occurs. The more often a story is repeated, the

more likely it will be twisted, and the sheer numbers of people involved will amplify the likelihood that the confidence will be breached.

Consider the stream of people through a patient's room on an average day in a large teaching hospital. Let us consider the case of a forty-seven-year-old man recovering from an acute myocardial infarction (heart attack) who has just been transferred from the coronary-care unit to the cardiac floor. These are some of the health care workers who might visit him in one day:

- the nursing assistant who changes his bed and helps him wash
- the medication nurse with his blood pressure pills
- a nursing instructor assigning patients for her students
- a student nurse doing research for tomorrow's assignment
- the head nurse
- the nursing supervisor
- a physiotherapist
- a respiratory therapist
- the dietitian
- his cardiologist
- the cardiologist's resident
- the cardiologist's intern
- a medical student assigned to take a medical history
- a social worker ...

The list continues on, and on depending upon the individual patient's problems. Each of these persons has legitimate access to the patient's chart, and they are only those directly involved in his care. Others such as the ward clerk, medical-record technicians, quality-assurance auditors, and even the business office also can have access. In fact, one physician reported doing a survey to determine how many people had access to one of his patient's charts and his count totalled seventy-five (Annas 1989). Do you know how many people have read your medical record lately?

An Overriding Public Interest

Finally, we come to the erosion factor that is alluded to in many of the others and is proving to be one of the most difficult for us as individuals to deal with. This is the need to consider the overriding public interest. In other words, sometimes the risks to the public are made greater by maintaining an individual's confidentiality than by breaking it. This illustrates a general trend in medical ethics today – namely, the movement away from the strictly patient-centred ethics of the Hippocratic tradition towards more concern for the greater good. This general inclination is evident in areas of society outside of medical practice as well. We have become increasingly concerned about how individual actions, often based on beliefs about freedom of choice, are having an impact on society. This is particularly evident in the area of environmental concerns.

Probably the highest profile of these concerns about patient confidentiality, and the one most hotly debated, relates to HIV carriers (those patients who carry the human immunodeficiency virus believed to cause AIDS). Some people have advocated that the seriousness of the infection makes it ethical for a physician to breach a patient's confidentiality if the patient refuses to tell those people who might be at risk of contracting the disease from him or her.

These factors, whether reasonable or unreasonable, have eroded what used to be considered a sacred trust in the doctor–patient relationship. Regardless of the validity of these transgressions, they have changed irrevocably the way we view our encounters with our physicians.

GENERAL EFFECTS OF THIS EROSION

The deterioration of the value of confidentiality in health care has had three general effects. Some are intentional; others are not.

The first of these problems originates with the doctor. If a physician believes that a private detail of a patient's condition might be a problem for the patient if it became known, he or she may knowingly neglect to make a record of it. Incomplete documentation on the chart could have far-reaching implications for care at a later date. The classic example occurs when a doctor in a small town chooses not to document a patient's complaint regarding something like spousal abuse or sexual dysfunction if he or she knows that the office nurse or clerk is a friend or relative of the patient. If the problem were to escalate later, this lack of documentation could be a problem for both the patient and the doctor. This is an example of a doctor's good intentions gone awry, doing the wrong thing for the right reasons.

The second effect of these erosions of patient confidentiality originates with the patient. If as a patient you fear that an intimate detail of your medical or relevant social condition might become public once you reveal it to your doctor, you may be hampering your physician's ability to give you the best possible medical advice and treatment. If, for example, a patient moves to a new state or province to take a new job and consults a new physician, he or she might choose to omit a detail or two of past medical history. If the patient suffered from epileptic seizures in the past and wished to take a driver's test in this new area without a lot of red tape, he or she might hide this information, thereby preventing the new doctor from relating it to the proper authorities in charge of issuing drivers' licences. A number of things could occur as a result. First, the patient or others might be hurt, or even killed, should a seizure occur while the patient is driving. Second, the patient will not be receiving proper follow-up for this previously diagnosed medical condition.

Finally, as an overall effect, the modern erosion of confidentiality in medical care is taking its toll on the trusting relationship between doctor and patient. You may find yourself trusting your doctor less because you are not certain how secret your secrets really are, and this may have a spill-over effect on your ability to trust this professional's advice and opinions. On the other hand, physicians may also trust their patients less, believing that crucial information may be being withheld. Since such failures to disclose information can hamper the physician in terms of ability to do his or her job properly, the doctor's fear of being sued increases, and the cycle of mistrust continues.

IMPROVING YOUR CONFIDENTIALITY QUOTIENT

While the previous discussion may lead you to believe that all is lost when it comes to your trusting relationship with a doctor today, this is not necessarily the case. An informed patient is an empowered patient, and you can do a number of things to inform yourself about the extent to which you should be worried about your secrets. Once you have a handle on the number of opportunities that exist for your confidentiality to be breached, you can do one of two things: (1) you can approach your physician about the problem areas and see that something is done about them, or (2) you can find a new doctor.

First, here is a series of questions which may help you to determine the extent to which your encounters with your physician are confidential.

Visits with your doctor:
- Does he or she always make sure that your discussions take place only in a private office, with the door closed?
- Does he or she take telephone calls in your presence, exposing the intimate details of other patients? (If you overhear a patient's call, you can bet that your next phone call may be overheard as well.)

Your medical record:
- Is your chart always kept closed unless someone is using it for a specific reason?
- Is access to the office file room restricted?
- Are unfiled documents such as laboratory reports and letters from consultants kept in closed files until reviewed? Are they then filed immediately?

Computer use:
- Is the computer screen visible only to the person using it?

- Does the computer operator always clear the screen after working with a record?

In order to answer some of these questions you will merely have to be more observant on your next visit to the doctor. To obtain answers to other questions, you will have to ask directly. If your doctor wants to know why you are asking, do not hesitate to tell him or her. You have a right to know how secure your medical secrets are (more about your rights in the next chapter).

It would be nice to be able to find a situation where the confidentiality of our medical information had improved rather than deteriorated. At least one such situation comes to mind. In the past, if your mother or father was diagnosed with a life-threatening illness, typically one such as cancer, the doctor might, in an attempt to 'protect' the patient, tell the 'next of kin' and not the patient. With today's climate of respect of the patient's right to know, this practice has changed. It is more common today for only the patient to be told, leaving it to his or her discretion who else is entitled to know.

WHAT YOU CAN DO

Obviously, in the world of medical care today, there is a need to strike a balance between absolute confidentiality for one individual patient and the needs of society at large. Since medical and other health professionals seem to be having such difficulty with this issue, you the consumer will have to do your part and help. Following from the questions above, here are some measures you might consider taking.

- Sit in your doctor's reception room and observe the extent to which people other than your doctor can view your medical records (either on a computer screen or in open files on the desk). If you are unsure about the security of their method, tell your doctor about your concerns.
- If you can hear what a staff member in your doctor's office is saying about another patient, approach that person and tell

him or her that you can overhear. If there is no change in behaviour, tell your doctor. If you observe this behaviour again in future, and you are concerned about it, perhaps you should consider a different doctor.

- If your doctor answers the telephone while you are in a consultation and begins to talk about another patient, ask him or her if you should leave. If he or she does not indicate that you should leave and continues to discuss confidential information, leave anyway and discuss this breach of confidentiality with the doctor later.
- Ask your doctor about accessibility of patient information within the office. For example, does he or she ever let people use patients' charts to gather data for studies?
- Tell your doctor how you feel about other members of your family having access to information about your medical condition. If there is a family member with whom you would like the doctor to speak, make this known. If you do not wish any other family members to be made privy to information about you, make this clear.
- If you are in a hospital elevator (or other location) and you overhear a conversation about an identifiable patient, politely inform those who are discussing the patient that you can overhear them and ask if they should be discussing patients in this way in public places.

5

Consenting to Treatment:
Do You Know What You Are Doing?

Knowledge is not lost by giving it to someone else, as happens with
other commodities. If I share information with you, you gain something and I lose nothing. (Ladd 1980)

Dr Goode's patient Mr Fiske was a forty-year-old who had come
to the office complaining of recurring indigestion. After a careful
physical examination, Dr Goode decided that Mr Fiske's pain
was probably caused by his heart. A very busy, stressed-out
businessman, Mr Fiske had all the classic risk factors. He was a
driven person, ate a diet high in fast-food fatty calories, had
smoked until just recently, and had borderline high blood pressure that Dr Goode had been monitoring for the past three years.
All in all, Dr Goode had often thought that Mr Fiske was a heart
attack looking for a place to happen. Now it was time to refer
this young man to a cardiologist, and Dr Goode knew just the
heart specialist to send him to.

Mr Fiske's first visit to the heart specialist involved a physical
examination, an electrocardiogram (a tracing of the electrical
conduction in his heart muscle), which a technician carried out;
and a stress test, during which he had to exert himself on a
treadmill while hooked up to an ECG machine. None of this
alarmed him very much, but on his second visit he was unpre-
pared for what the cardiologist, Dr MacGregor, had to say.

'Mr Fiske, I'm afraid the results of your stress test are very
worrisome. It seems you have quite severe myocardial insuffi-

ciency. I want you to have a cardiac cath ... I need your signature on this consent form, and then I'll send it over to the hospital with the requisition and we'll get you settled.'

He pulled a form out of his desk drawer. 'You've no doubt heard of a cardiac cath. We do them all the time.'

Mr Fiske knew that he had heard the term before, but he had been so sure that the doctor would tell him that he just had the makings of an ulcer that the idea of heart disease knocked the wind out of him. He didn't know quite how to respond.

Dr MacGregor evidently took his silence as agreement that he had, indeed, heard of a cardiac cath before.

'We'll be inserting the catheter into your femoral artery and passing it through your abdominal aorta to your heart. When it reaches your heart, we'll inject a radiopaque dye through the catheter so that we'll be able to visualize clearly the areas of stenosis. You don't have any allergies do you?'

Mr Fiske shook his head slightly. Dr MacGregor continued his monologue.

'There is a small risk that the catheter could irritate the electrical conduction system of your heart as it passes through, thus setting off an arrhythmia, but that's unlikely. We do thousands of these every year. Haven't lost one yet.' He chuckled. 'Do you have any questions before you sign the consent for the procedure?'

Any questions? Mr Fiske was still back at the part about threading a catheter and injecting his heart. And what exactly did the doctor mean by the term 'small risk'? And what would happen if they found 'areas of stenosis'? The problem was that Mr Fiske was too dumbfounded by the news that he needed this procedure to even know what to ask first. He took the pen Dr MacGregor handed to him and signed the form.

Did Dr MacGregor satisfy the requirements for having the patient give informed consent to this invasive procedure? To his mind, he probably did. Did Mr Fiske make an informed decision? Hardly.

The concept of informed consent is the main hallmark of what is today's patient autonomy, the right to control your own care and make your own decisions. If you are to have control over your health care, then it stands to reason that the decisions made, including what diagnostic procedures and treatments to have, and when, as well as those not to have, have to be made by you, an informed health care consumer. Your ability to make such decisions depends on three things: how well informed you are and what you understand this information to mean to you; whether you are competent to give consent; and the extent to which you are giving this consent voluntarily. Before we get to that, however, we'll examine the development of this concept in modern medical care and find out how doctors are handling it today.

'INFORMED CONSENT' YESTERDAY AND TODAY

While we prefer to call this 'informed decision making,' the term 'informed consent' is the one that physicians usually use. The problem with the term 'consent' is that it can be interpreted in a number of ways, not all of which are useful to you when making these decisions. While it can mean 'voluntary agreement,' it can also refer to 'voluntary yielding,' 'acquiescence or even 'compliance.' This concept of 'voluntary yielding' has further implications in that it suggests that one person gives in to the will of another. When it comes to patients 'consenting' to medical treatment, we would like to think that this is never the case. We shall see.

Historically, the idea of the patient having a say in how medical care and treatment are provided is an early twentieth-century phenomenon. In 1905, while making assertions about a patient's right to inviolability of his [sic] person, one judge said that this right forbids a doctor to violate the bodily integrity of a person without consent (Pratt v. Davis, 1905).

Legal precedents in the United States at the beginning of this century provided early guidance, but it was not until 1957 that the term *informed consent* was coined in the California Court of Appeal (Silverman 1989). The case involved a patient who had suffered permanent paralysis following a surgical procedure.

This patient claimed that the physicians were negligent by failing to inform him that there was a risk of paralysis with this procedure. The judge's deliberations resulted in what was referred to as 'a new duty of disclosure, tempered with discretion.' This phrase refers to the doctor's responsibility to use good judgment in giving the patient all the necessary information. The judge used the term 'informed consent' and it has stuck.

Today, in every hospital and clinic across the continent, medical consent forms are a standard paper item. How they are used, however, varies considerably.

Dr Jay Katz, professor of law, medicine, and psychiatry at Yale University, has written that doctors have embraced the concept of patient autonomy and informed consent with nothing more than mechanical observance. He believes that their chief motivation is not decision-making partnerships with patients, but an attempt to avoid being sued (Katz 1992).

It seems, then, that our story of the cardiologist going through the motions of providing adequate information to a patient so that the patient may make an informed decision is probably not far from the realities of many doctor–patient encounters.

If this view does, indeed, represent how many doctors feel about informing patients and making them part of the overall medical decision-making process, it does not speak very highly of doctors' respect for their patients. Fortunately, not everyone agrees with Dr Katz. In fact, many doctors, those coming through current medical school programs in particular, welcome your input and seek it out. Even if a doctor does not seek it out, however, that does not mean that he or she would not appreciate it if you took the initiative.

THE 'PROPERLY' INFORMED PATIENT

One of the significant and recurring problems that physicians have in supporting initiatives that lead to patient control harkens back to the power imbalance in the relationship that you have with your doctor. You need information. Your doctor either has that information or has access to it, and you rely on him or her to give it you. That puts the doctor in a position of power relative to you. Further complicating the issue is the fact that even doctors who truly believe in developing partnerships with patients may lack the communication skills necessary to provide you with the information you need at a level that you can understand.

Physician and ethicist Howard Brody (1989, 5) says this: 'Informed consent, properly understood, must be considered an essential ingredient of good patient care, and a physician who lacks the skills to inform patients appropriately and obtain proper consent should be viewed as lacking in essential medical skills necessary for practice. It is not enough to see informed consent as a nonmedical, legalistic exercise ...'

A doctor's lack of communication skills, then, is no different from his or her lack of ability to carry out any other necessary medical procedure. As a patient you have the right to expect an adequate level of communication skills.

In our search to be truly informed decision makers in our own health care, is it possible to be overinformed? We have already suggested that there are significant problems associated with being underinformed, but is the opposite just as problematic in its own way? It has been suggested that possibly a lot of new information, coupled with inappropriate communication methods, can lead to patients' being too terrified to truly comprehend what the doctor is saying. As a result the patient is unable to make an informed decision. This stress can be lessened to some extent by a physician who knows you, the patient, well enough to be able to determine how much information to give you at one time and has enough experience to be able to provide it to you in a way that is not as likely to terrify you quite as much. Not all doctors are able to do this.

The Canadian Medical Association's policy on informed decision making states clearly that the doctor's duty to provide all the appropriate information to the patient 'does not extend to giving the patient frightening or distressing information' (Canadian Medical Association 1986). It leaves the decision of who is likely to be frightened by what information up to the clinical judgment of the individual physician. Thus, just as capability in clinical judgment varies, so too will the decisions of physicians to either give you information or withhold it from you.

There is another important concern that you should consider in ensuring that you are truly exercising your right to make an informed decision: Whose responsibility is it to inform you and actually obtain consent? This is a problem in many medical institutions today. Should someone who is not actually doing a procedure on you provide you with information and obtain your signature on a legally binding form? In other words, is it ethical for your doctor, for example, to send in a nurse, a technician or an intern to get your signature for a procedure that will be performed by yet another person? Some would argue that a nurse might possibly have more highly developed communication skills than a particular doctor, but it is still that physician who should be talking to you. It might help if the nurse were present so that she or he might follow up, but the responsibility is still the physician's.

What can you do if you do not believe that you have been properly informed?

- First, do not sign anything.
- Enlist the help of a family member, a friend, or even a member of the nursing staff to help you to develop a list of questions that you need answered.
- If you still do not feel comfortable with your understanding of the information provided by the doctor, get another doctor.

GIVING YOUR CONSENT VOLUNTARILY

Along with the requirement that you be properly informed in order to be able to give consent, you must also be giving it voluntarily. You should not feel that you are being coerced, however gently, into making a decision. It is your right to make this decision, free from any outside pressure. If you have sufficient information and are competent to give the consent, then pressure from an outside source can only place stress on you.

Where might this coercion originate? The most common place from which this undue influence arises is from your doctor, who likely believes that he or she is only doing what is best for you. The following true story illustrates coercion that is difficult to see at first glance.

In the early 1980s, a group of well-intentioned health professionals produced a videotape that was designed to persuade people to donate organs for transplantation. While the film has some merits, it contains a segment that is of particular concern.

On camera, a doctor from a transplant program relates a story of one particular patient who, following an accident, was lying in a coma in an intensive care unit, brain dead. The neurosurgeon caring for this young man had approached his family to ask if they would consent to removal of their son's organs for transplant, and they had refused this consent. The director of the hospital's transplant program then informed the surgeon that he would like to talk to the family so that they might be apprised of all the facts. He proceeded to tell the family about how much life was left in 'that wonderful young body' and that he was 'perfectly alive except that his brain is gone.' Apart from the obvious concern about telling the family that there is still life there, the problem of consent was yet to come.

The doctor then went on to tell the family about a patient 'upstairs whose heart is dying hour by hour but whose brain is very much alive' and that the transplant team could 'retrieve life from him and transfer it to her.' Regardless of how noble one might believe this act of donating organs after death is, in this instance subtle pressure is being placed on a grieving family who are made to feel even a little bit responsible for the life of that other person. This is dangerous, but it does illustrate the nature of the subtleties of coercion in health care decision making.

Another situation that is probably even more common is the physician's approach to obtaining consent through the offer of a reward. This occurs primarily when the consent that is being sought is for you to take part in some kind of research and is more of a problem when the research is based in a doctor's office than when it is hospital-based as hospitals usually have a review committee to determine the ethics of research studies. The most common kind of research in such situations is a drug trial (more about these in chapter 17). If a doctor is working with a drug company to test a drug that is already on the market, the inducement is likely that you will receive the drug free of charge during the period of the research. Considering the cost of drugs today, such an offer can be very enticing. While the potential harm to you in this situation is probably minimal, you might be required to submit to tests, and when the trial ends you could be left on a drug which might be considerably more expensive than your present one.

Clearly, you must be allowed to make your own decision without undue pressure from health professionals, however well-meaning they might be.

THE CONCEPT OF COMPETENCE

The third requirement for your consent to be valid in health care is that you must be *competent* to give that consent. This seems clear enough, but the definition and determination of competence are not at all simple in some situations.

The question of competence in medical care is a little like that of innocence in the justice system: you are considered to be competent until proven otherwise. In legal situations it may be useful to consider competence as an all-or-nothing situation: either you are competent to make your own decision or you are not. In health care, however, we recognize that there are degrees of competence, and these can change over and time and can fluctuate with the course of an illness (Cahn 1980). In fact, from a medical perspective, the loss of competence to give consent for medical diagnosis and treatment is not a black-and-white declaration from the outset. A person may actually be incompetent one day and competent the next, depending upon the cause of the problem.

As a health care consumer, you cannot take this notion of competence to give consent lightly. If someone is declared incompetent under the law, the consequences are far-reaching and go beyond decisions about health care. In some areas, for example, once you are declared incompetent, you are no longer permitted to drive a car, manage your own finances, or even vote.

How, then, is competence determined in health care? The biggest problem here is that there is no universally accepted definition of competence in this area. There is no standard, objective test that all doctors can apply in these situations. There are simply vague guidelines, and a lot of subjectivity. In a position paper prepared for the Canadian Psychiatric Association, the author set out four questions that physicians should pose in determining a patient's capacity to consent. The answers to the following questions should be 'yes':

1. Does the patient understand the condition for which the treatment is proposed?
2. Does the patient understand the nature and purpose of the treatment?
3. Does the patient understand the risks and benefits involved in undergoing the treatment?
4. Does the patient understand the risks and benefits involved in *not* undergoing the treatment? (Cahn 1980, 81)

While in theory these may be useful guidelines for doctors, they are difficult to interpret without subjectivity creeping into the discussion. There have been cases of doctors seeking to have patients declared incompetent so that they may go ahead with whatever medical procedure they deem to be in the best interests of the patient. Some of the highest-profile cases have involved individuals with certain religious beliefs that prevent them from consenting to the advised treatment. Other cases have involved doctors, believing they know best, failing to understand that patients bring to the doctor–patient encounter a whole different set of values than the one they possess.

It is difficult, for example, for a young physician, trained to fight death as the enemy, to understand that someone could choose to refuse life-saving treatment. This young doctor may honestly believe that no competent person who truly understands the risks and benefits could possibly refuse. The logical extension for that physician is that this lack of understanding indicates incompetence. For the patient who is refusing the offered treatment, convincing this doctor of patient competence can be difficult. It is even more difficult to convince the doctor if the patient's family fails to understand and advocate on his or her behalf. Sometimes it is the relatives who wish to have members of their families declared incompetent so that their own wishes may take precedence over those of the patient. This can be an especially troublesome problem for older patients.

Before we examine a standard consent form that a hospital may ask you to sign for a procedure, you may be interested in some guidelines that have been given to doctors. These 'maxims' suggest to physicians the following:

• Tell your patients all they want and need to know about their medical care.
• Know your own expertise as a physician and do not hesitate to refer patients to more qualified colleagues.
• Listen closely to your patients and, if necessary, their families and acquaintances in order to determine what is in their best interests.
• Aim for agreement with your patients as to the best medical treatment for them.
• Where agreement is absent, defer to your patients' judgement except where their competence is doubtful or lacking. (Royal College of Physicians and Surgeons of Canada 1987)

TOURING A CONSENT FORM

A standard hospital consent form (see figure 5.1) usually contains four short sections.

Figure 5.1
Standard Consent to Diagnostic, Operative or Treatment Procedures

1. I authorize Dr _____ (attending physician) and other such medical personnel or staff as they may in their discretion select or approve of to act or assist them under their supervision and direction, to perform the following diagnostic, operative, or treatment procedure _____upon me or_____ _____(relationship) with any of the following limitations:

_____

_____

2. The nature of what is proposed as well as the risks involved have been explained to me by Dr _____ (informing physician or physicians) and I understand them. All of my questions regarding the procedure have been answered.

3. I also consent to such additional or alternative procedures as in the opinion of the medical staff performing the procedure mentioned above are considered immediately necessary and vital to the health of _____.

4. I agree to the retention by hospital staff (for the purpose of diagnosis) or the disposal of any material that may be removed during the diagnostic, operative, or treatment procedure.

DATED this ____ day of _____, 19____ at ____ hours

_____   _____
Signature of patient or alternative   Signature of physician

_____
Signature of witness (if required)

(Optional part)
I confirm that I have explained the nature, expected results and significant risks involved in this procedure to the patient named above.

DATE _____ PHYSICIAN _____

1. Section 1 indicates the name of the attending physician and states exactly what investigation, treatment, or operative procedure this particular consent is for. Especially in teaching hospitals, this section also indicates that you are consenting to have other medical personnel or staff that this physician might select either to act under his or her supervision or to assist. If you sign a form which states this, a resident, intern, or medical student who is deemed by your attending physician to be competent to do the procedure under supervision will have your permission to proceed.

2. Section 2 indicates that you have been properly informed, and who did the informing. It should not allow for any name other than a physician's to appear here. It should state that you are satisfied that your questions have been answered and that you understand what will be done. If you have not been properly informed, do not sign it.

3. Section 3 is the one that often gives patients cause to pause and reflect. It usually states that you are also consenting to any additional or alternative procedures that, in the opinion of your attending physician, are immediately necessary. In other words, for example, if they find something that they were not expecting, they will have permission to go ahead and treat it. Giving this permission could be very useful for you. It might spare you from another surgery, or it could even save your life. On the other hand, you may not want to consent to anything other than the specified procedure or treatment. If you are having a breast biopsy, you may not wish to consent to having them carry on with a mastectomy without letting you know the results of the biopsy, even though the delay that occurs may lead to the need for a second anaesthetic. You may, however, trust your physician to make certain decisions for you, and consent beforehand to other procedures if certain events are encountered.

4. Section 4, optional on some forms, refers to your consent to have any material removed from you during the procedure (e.g., tumours) either retained by the hospital for diagnostic purposes or disposed of. It is not the business of the hospital to return these to you.

5. Hospital consent forms must be signed by the physician, the patient, and a witness. In the case where the patient is unable to provide consent (a child, an unconscious person), the next of kin is approached for consent.

Hospitals have made great strides in their attempt to ensure that patients are truly informed about procedures before they consent to them. Some have even produced videotapes that explain some common types of procedures, and arrange for both a nurse and a physician to answer questions. Often, however, it may seem that securing your consent is simply a matter of avoiding a lawsuit. Whatever their motivation, it is in your best interests to avail yourself of all opportunities to be more informed about your care and to play an active role in the decision making.

WHAT YOU CAN DO

There are several actions that you, the patient, can take to play your part in being properly informed to make appropriate decisions for you. You, too, have responsibilities.

- Seek out information on health and medical issues that affect you directly or indirectly. For example, if you have a complaint that you present to your doctor and he or she begins to investigate it, seek out information. Contact the local office of a related non-profit organization such as the American or Canadian Cancer Society, the Heart and Stroke Foundation or Heart Association, or the Alzheimer Society. There are organizations that are devoted to most major and some not-so-major medical conditions. Most of them provide literature written for the layperson.
- When you are faced with a major decision, as we mentioned earlier, you might consider enlisting the assistance of a trusted family member or a friend. This person may be able to help you to think of questions to ask or angles to explore. A degree of distance from the problem is often helpful.

- If a doctor or nurse explains something to you and you do not understand, be very clear about this. Most of them are only too happy to help you further once they are aware of your confusion. Avoid nodding your head in agreement when you really are unsure of the meaning and implications of what you are being told.

6

Patients' Rights/Doctors' Rights ...
Never the Twain Shall Meet?

When you enter the health care system, you enter a world over which
you have little or no control, in which you meekly follow orders.
    At best it's a humiliating experience. At worst, it's a life-threatening
one. Your only defense is your rights as a consumer.
– Charles Inlander and Eugene I. Pavalon, *Your Medical Rights* (1990, 9)

If the number of health care activist groups that have begun to
spring up all over North America is any indication, the idea of
patients' rights is certainly timely. Along with concerns for
human rights, women's rights, minority rights, and all the other
rights movements of the twentieth century, the issue of patients'
rights has come into its own as consumer groups fight to take
back control of their health care decisions. For members of the
medical profession, the notion of patients having rights can be
viewed either as a welcome addition to their decision making or
as a nuisance of no small proportions.

    Health care is a consumable service. Thus any rights that you
have as a consumer can be claimed when you take on the role of
patient. Although the consumerist movement in North America
is widely perceived to be a child of the 1960s and Ralph Nader,
its roots go back to the late nineteenth century. The National
Consumers League, established in 1899, is a consumerist land-
mark that continues to find support almost a century later
(Mayer 1989; Sorenson 1978).

    In the 1960s, however, the movement seemed to take off. It

was given a shot in the arm when John F. Kennedy declared that consumers have four basic rights:

1. the right to safety
2. the right to choose
3. the right to be heard
4. the right to be informed.

These are rights that health care consumers also have. With this as a given, there are several questions that need to be answered about rights:

- To what extent are patients' rights respected in medical care today?
- Do doctors' rights have any effect on encounters with patients?
- What happens when a patient's rights conflict with those of another patient?
- What happens when a patient's rights conflict with the doctor's rights?

Before we can determine how the medical establishment handles these ethical problems, however, we must first establish what rights really are from an ethical perspective. Then we need to examine how doctors define those rights in practice.

WHAT IS A RIGHT?

We use the word 'rights' daily. It seems to slide easily off our tongues and the tongues of every journalist in North America. But we often fail to stop long enough to consider whether or not we are all talking about the same thing. What are rights, and where do they come from? What do they mean for you as a health care consumer? And, even more important, what are their limits?

Rights are claims that we make on other people and on society and, more important than this, they are *justified claims*. How claims are justified varies with the right at issue. For example, we say that everyone has a right to a fair trial. This legal right is a justified claim because we have a law to warrant it. When you are talking about moral rights, however, you have entered into territory that is much more open to interpretation, primarily because members of North American society, which is heterogeneous in nature, do not share the same morality or justify the same claims.

There are three things that we need to keep in mind about rights:

- A right is something that you *choose* to exercise or not; no one can force you to act upon a claim that you make. In other words, you can choose to give up a right. If you decide that, for any one of a number of reasons, you are not prepared to exercise your right to make health care decisions for yourself, you may give up that right to someone else.
- Doctors and other health professionals have a duty to uphold your rights. Since it is our accepted convention today that competent patients have the right to choose for themselves their course of medical treatment, doctors have a duty to ensure that they can exercise this right and have no right to interfere with this claim.
- A claim that you make, even if it can be justified, is not a right if you do not have access to it. It would be inappropriate for us to suggest that everyone who needs a heart transplant has a right to one since there will not be enough transplantable hearts available to fulfil the duties inherent in that right. On the other hand, if society decides that everyone has a right to a minimum standard of care, society has a responsibility to ensure that this can, indeed, be a right by making it accessible to everyone.

It may be apparent by now that there is another concept that goes hand in hand with rights – namely, responsibility. With every right comes a responsibility. For every justified claim that is made, another person or persons have a duty to uphold that right. There is also another way of looking at the relationship between rights and responsibilities: if you have a specific right, then you also have a responsibility not to abuse that right. Before we discuss your responsibilities, though, we need to identify just what rights we are talking about.

WHAT RIGHTS DO PATIENTS HAVE?

It might seem to you that patients' rights in the health care systems of North America today must to be obvious to everyone, and that they are undeniable. This is a misconception. While some rights seem fairly self-evident, the fact is that there is considerable disagreement about exactly what rights patients do have, and about what doctors and other health professionals can do to see that these are upheld. That patients and doctors have disagreed about their rights from time to time is evident from the proliferation of patients' rights and consumer health care groups.

With its head office in California, the National Health Federation is one of the oldest patients' rights organizations in North America. Since its founding in 1955, the federation, which refers to itself as 'a non-profit, consumer-oriented organization devoted exclusively to health matters,' has had the mandate to advocate for 'the absolute right of the people to enjoy the civil liberty of freedom of choice in matters of personal health where such choices do not infringe upon the liberties of others' (NHF Silver Anniversary Booklet 1970).

Other such organizations exist that advocate for specific rights of health care consumers. The People's Medical Society is another, perhaps higher-profile, patients' rights organization, based in Allentown, Pennsylvania. Their impressive board of directors includes people who hold such positions as professor at the Yale University School of Medicine and director general of the Health Promotion Directorate of Health and Welfare Canada. The high profile this group has achieved comes primarily as a result of the publications that have been produced by its members. These include books such as *Medicine on Trial: The Appall-*

ing *Story of Ineptitude, Malfeasance, Neglect and Arrogance* (Inlander, Levin, and Weiner 1988) and more recently *Your Medical Rights: How to Become an Empowered Consumer* (Inlander and Pavalon 1990).

According to their promotional literature, the People's Medical Society exists to fulfil the following objectives: 'to give people the information they need to protect themselves in their daily lives' and 'to bring thousands of people together as a social and political force strong enough to stand up to the medical establishment.' It seems, then, that thousands of people do perceive a need to stand up to the medical establishment.

Here is a brief summary of the patients' rights as the consumer activist groups see them. As a patient, you have a right to:

- be treated with respect and dignity and have your immediate family treated with respect. This respect may be as simple as not being referred to by your first name by a doctor or nurse;
- receive a reasonable response to requests for services;
- receive humane and efficient care;
- receive safe care;
- receive reasonable continuity of care. This can be a particular problem if you are being treated in a hospital clinic situation. Seeing a different doctor and/or nurse every time you visit is disruptive to the therapeutic relationship that you should be developing with a caregiver;
- be informed of a health professional's morality if this may affect treatment. If you are seeking counselling for unwanted pregnancy, you have a right to know that this doctor is a staunch pro-life supporter as his or her advice may be significantly affected by this moral stance;
- adequate information about your disease. This means that you have a right not only to be given such information but to have it tailored to your level of understanding. You have the right to ask questions and expect that those questions will be answered;
- choose your own medical therapy. This right can be exercised only if all the requirements that we discussed in chapter 5 are

met – that is, you are adequately informed, you are competent to choose, you are able to choose freely, and the treatment is available;
- not be subjected to unnecessary diagnostic procedures. A competent physician should be able to select appropriate diagnostic procedures based on your medical history. Except in very mysterious circumstances, the shotgun approach to diagnosis, usually embarked upon by a doctor who fears being sued, is a violation of your rights;
- not be emotionally exploited;
- privacy. Now that you are familiar with what the concept of confidentiality in health care means to both doctors and patients, you need to know that it is a right that health professionals have a duty to uphold;
- a second opinion. There is no requirement for you to accept what any one doctor has to say about your medical condition. In this case, the doctor has a duty to assist you with obtaining that second opinion if necessary or, at the very least, to accept your decision gracefully;
- death with dignity. Know that you have this right. In chapter 16 we will discuss what this can mean to you.

Your rights as a patient are violated as a result of a number of problems, including persistent medical paternalism (the father-knows-best attitude) and the fact that conflicts develop between the rights of one individual patient and those of another individual patient, between an individual patient and the rights of society, and between the rights of the patient and the rights of the doctor. First, we'll look at the rights that doctors have.

WHAT RIGHTS DOES THE DOCTOR HAVE?

Western society is committed to upholding human rights. Both the U.S. and the Canadian constitutions provide protection under the law for human rights. Thus, since physicians are human, they do, indeed, have rights. While this may be fairly straightforward, what is less clear is what those rights are in the context of their relationships with you, their patients.

It seems that organized medicine in North America had the idea of the rights of physicians in mind from a very early stage. When the Canadian Medical Association had its first meeting, in early September 1868, their Committee on Medical Ethics presented its Code of Medical Ethics, which was based heavily on the American Medical Association's Code of Ethics adopted in 1847. The final article indicates the obligations of the public to the physician (from which we can infer the physician's rights in relation):

The benefits accruing to the public, directly and indirectly, from the active and unwearied beneficence of the profession, are so numerous and important, that physicians are justly entitled to the utmost consideration and respect from the community. The public ought likewise to entertain a just appreciation of medical qualification ... (Canadian Medical Association 1868)

It seems quite clear from the above that physicians, at least those in the latter part of the nineteenth century, believed that they have a right to respect from their patients. If you consider that each of us as a human being has a right to be treated with respect, then this is certainly true. If, on the other hand, you believe that respect is not a right, but rather something to be earned, this article in the medical code of ethics is presumptuous at best. Based on today's medical standards, doctors' credentials do not automatically entitle them to any respect that they have not earned. Respect is based on competence, compassion, and an ability to recognize and deal with ethical dilemmas.

There are, however, some specific rights that physicians of the late twentieth century claim. Three of these are the doctor's right to:

1. refuse to treat any given patient;
2. maintain his or her own privacy; and
3. preserve the safety of his or her person.

All of these claims can pose problems for the health care consumer.

The issue of a doctor's right to refuse to treat a patient has fuelled many heated debates between physicians and advocacy groups. Most physicians today believe that they have a right to refuse to treat any given patient except in an emergency situation. This claim is also justified by professional codes of ethics of doctors that state clearly that this is a doctor's right. It seems, then, a doctor can refuse to treat you for any reason at all and has no obligation to explain him or herself to you. It may be that his or her practice is full and there is no room for another patient; the doctor may not feel competent to treat your specific condition; the doctor may not want to treat your specific condition; the doctor may not like the colour of your skin, your sexual orientation, and on and on. An individual doctor's justification for this refusal may be very personal and he or she is not obliged to explain it to you. The bottom line is that doctors reserve this right to restrict access to their personal practices.

Predictably, this stance is not always popular. Although it is generally accepted that, once a physician enters into a relationship with a patient – and this is supported by the codes of ethics of the medical associations of both Canada and the United States – that doctor has a duty to treat the patient to the best of his or her ability. There is, however, no requirement that a doctor enter into a relationship with any given patient. It has been argued that being required to accept all would-be patients could interfere with a given patient's right to be treated.

The second claim, the doctor's right to maintain personal privacy, was a given for many years but, again, as we approach the end of the twentieth century, it is also being disputed hotly. Just as some issues have threatened your medical confidentiality, some situations have created controversy over the limits of privacy for individual doctors. This has come to a head mostly as a result of the AIDS concerns of today.

At this point in the history of the human immunodeficiency virus, the organism believed to cause AIDS, there has been only one publicly known incident of an HIV-positive health professional transmitting the virus to a patient, although there have now been many others who have become known to be HIV-positive. The situation involved Dr David Acer, a Florida dentist who allegedly infected a number of patients before his death in 1990 of an AIDS-related illness. In 1991, Kimberly Bergalis, one of those patients whom he infected, was in living-rooms all across the continent as she appeared, near death, before a U.S. congressional committee to plead the case for mandatory HIV testing for health professionals. She was unsuccessful in this attempt and died of AIDS-related illness in December 1992, at the age of twenty-three.

Although this was a very moving case, and the medical associations of both the United States and Canada have examined this issue carefully, they still do not support the concept of either mandatory HIV screening for doctors or mandatory disclosure of their HIV-positive status. In July 1991, the U.S. Centers for Disease Control issued guidelines that indicated that doctors and other health professionals who are aware that they are HIV-positive should refrain from performing 'exposure-prone' procedures unless they have received expert guidance regarding specific circumstances under which they could do so (Dunn 1992). The term 'exposure-prone' has never been defined, and the medical associations cite lack of scientific evidence and catastrophic career repercussions as sufficient evidence to uphold the doctor's right to privacy.

The third claim that bears some consideration is that of physicians to the right to safety of person. While this may seem self-evident – that we all have this right, and, indeed, we have already stated that it is a right of each patient – its modern interpretation is the problem. It used to be that the doctor's main concern about safety of person was related to safety from assault by violent psychiatric patients. Today, as in the pre-antibiotic era, the physician is more likely to be concerned about assault from unseen sources – namely, micro-organisms. This right translates into a doctor's claim that he or she has a right to know about the HIV, hepatitis, and any other relevant status of any patient who comes for consultation. As you can see, these claims of rights on the parts of both doctors and patients can conflict. It is this area of conflict that results in some of the most pressing ethical dilemmas in health care today. As one physician put it: 'There are many rights to be balanced, and no one interest group, either health care professionals or patients, has a monopoly on them. Destructive antagonism and lack of information are obstacles to reciprocity' (McQueen 1992, 301).

CONFLICTING RIGHTS ...

Ever since Hippocrates began teaching his patient-centred approach to medicine 2,400 years ago, physicians have been attempting to do good and to do no harm. What do they do, then, when the good that they do for one (upholding one person's rights) does harm to another (violating his or her rights)?

Although there is no universally accepted way of deciding whose rights take precedence when there is a conflict, doctors must make these decisions every day in practice (whether they realize it or not). They use a variety of methods to make such determinations. Some of the questions they consider include:

• Are the claims that both parties are making really rights that are justified in some way?
• Why is each of these people claiming a right? What is the motivation of each?
• How important is each of the claims?
• If each claim were exercised, what would happen? Is one outcome more important than the other?
• Are these outcomes real or are they only possibilities?
• Does one of the claims have more benefit for larger numbers of people?
• What would happen if one or the other of the claims were not exercised?

Although these questions do not lead to a definitive choice, they do provide doctors with decisions that they can defend.

In the grey areas of medical ethics, this is often the best we can do.

WHAT YOU CAN DO

- In today's often complex world of medical decision making and your rights within that process, one of the most useful things that you can do is to recognize that you do, indeed, have rights, but that others have rights as well. Those others who have rights include both other health care consumers and your medical caregivers.
- Know your medical rights, but temper your demands within the context of what you know that your caregivers are capable of providing, given the circumstances. If, for example, you believe that you have a right to a certain type of medical treatment such as a transplant, you may be making unreasonable demands on your doctor to expect that a donor organ will become available for you.
- If you are in hospital and you feel that your rights have been neglected, you may be able to use the services of the hospital's patient advocate or ombudsperson. Ask the nurses if one is available.
- If you are dealing with a doctor in his or her private office and you feel your rights are not being respected, call the local medical association or medical licensing board to report your concerns.

7

And Justice for All ...

Allocating Scarce Resources

Dr Goode sighed as he looked at the appointment sheet on his desk. He had just returned from lunch and was preparing himself for a busy afternoon of seeing patients when he noticed the first name on the list. He knew why Mr White was here again. Six months ago, Mr White, a sixty-two-year-old with a long history of chest pain, had come to the office complaining of intense pain shooting down his arm. From all appearances, he was suffering from a heart attack, which was later confirmed when he was hastily admitted to the hospital via the emergency department. While he was in hospital, he had been told that what he really needed was triple coronary-artery bypass surgery, and he had agreed to go ahead with it.

There was, however, a major hitch in the plan for surgery: the public hospital had a surgical waiting-list for those with heart disease that is not immediately life-threatening. Mr White's condition was getting progressively worse, and he had come today to again ask Dr Goode if there was anything he could do to get him higher up on the list. Dr Goode knew that the only way for Mr White to get the surgery any time soon was to become moribund – in other words, to approach death from his disease. In private, Dr Goode had often wondered if his older patients were made to wait longer than his younger ones, but it was not a topic that was openly discussed in medical circles. He knew that he could do little more today than try to ease Mr White's worries about his long wait.

If most of the decisions that medical practitioners face today involved choices between something that is clearly evil and something that is clearly good, there would be no ethical dilemmas. The answers would be obvious. A dilemma, by its nature, involves hard choices, ones that require a selection of either the lesser of two evils or the greater of two conflicting goods. Nowhere is this more apparent than in the high-profile area of allocating scarce resources.

The idea that health care resources are in scarce supply and that decisions must be made about who gets what should be very troublesome for all of us as consumers. There are two uncomfortable questions that need answers:

• How can good decisions be made about who should get what in health care?
• Who should be making those decisions?

Much has been written about both of these questions, and no good answers have come to light that doctors, governments, allied health professionals, and, most important, health care consumers can agree upon. Whether people want to believe it or not, allocation decisions are made every day across this continent and, more than any other group involved in health care delivery, doctors make those decisions. How can we be certain those decisions are sound?

WHAT'S THE PROBLEM?

There is little doubt that if we continue to use health care resources at the rate we have been using them in the recent past, very soon there will not be enough to go around. There is a good argument to be made that this is already the case.

Today, health care in the United States costs well over $600 billion, and in Canada, with one-tenth the population, over $60 billion per year. As health-care consumers, however, we seem to think that we have a right to whatever medical science has to offer. As one Harvard law professor has said: 'If we commit ourselves to the notion that there is a right to whatever health care might be available, we become involved in a difficult situation whereby the overall national expenditure on health care will reach absurd proportions' (Fried 1977, 69). That was 1977, and that absurdity is creeping ever closer.

Although health care consumers' demands have fuelled what has become known as the overuse of health care resources, health professionals themselves, and doctors in particular, are largely to blame for the overuse that has led us to where we are today. It is widely believed that doctors are responsible for 70 to 80 per cent of all personal medical expenditures (Parsons 1985).

The first way that doctors contribute to this problem themselves is through their modern devotion to the technological fix. They have developed the habit of gambling on expensive, high-tech solutions that have not been adequately tested for value. Add on to this point of view the enormous media play that technology receives and you are left with doctors who are pressuring themselves and being pressured by their patients. Mammography is a good example. Despite evidence that indicates there is little or no benefit from this procedure for low-risk women under the age of fifty, many doctors continue to promote it. This issue is further complicated when much of the mammography equipment is owned by the physicians themselves and the question of paying for the equipment is of concern. As critics of modern medical technology have said: 'In their desire to do everything possible to help their patients, doctors often succumb to the terrible pressure to take action ... they jump the gun in advance of any good evidence to show their intervention will help, and wind up doing more harm than good, or wasting their time' (Rachlis and Kushner 1989, 59). Given current pressures on the health care system, good intentions are hardly a convincing argument for the validity of a medical approach. Doctors need a better reason than that to treat you.

The issue of doctors owning the major equipment to which they refer patients for tests or treatments is an interesting commentary on medical ethics, resource allocation, and free enterprise. Most physicians seem to think that, by owning the equipment, they can provide patients with better access, and that there will be more to go around. To test this theory, one enterprising doctor in California decided to conduct a mini-survey of access to magnetic resonance imaging (MRI). Orange County in California is privileged to have forty-one MRI centres. To put this in perspective, consider that there are 2.4 million residents and 798 square miles in Orange County. Canada, with 27 million residents and 4 million square miles, had twenty-two MRI centres at the time of the reported investigation. The doctor randomly called seventeen of the free-standing (not affiliated with hospitals) MRI centres, posing as three different patients. When he posed as an insured patient with a minor problem, the longest wait he encountered was forty-eight hours. When he posed as a medicaid patient with a possible brain tumour, six of the centres would give an appointment in two or three weeks if a personal physician would do the paperwork involved in getting payment. When he posed as an uninsured patient without cash, none of the seventeen centres would make an appointment (Morgan 1993).

Coronary-artery bypass graft surgery has come under increasing attack over the past few years, based on the belief that this expensive surgical procedure is done far too frequently on far too many people who would do just a well on more conservative treatment. One study reported in the *Journal of the American Medical Association* in 1988 indicated that as many as 50 per cent of all bypasses done in the United States are, at the very least, done for equivocal reasons or are totally inappropriate (Winslow and colleagues 1988). And other studies have lent credence to these results by following the subsequent progress of patients who either sought a second opinion and were encouraged to forgo the surgery or refused the surgery outright.

Health economists have suggested that a health care system that is doctor-driven rather than consumer-driven is more expensive to run, given the current love affair that the medical profession is having with technology (Ramsay 1991). Doctors are likely to disagree with this argument, taking the position that they might not be as likely to use all the high-tech gadgets if the media did not hype them to consumers so much, thereby making the system, at least to some extent, consumer-driven. This argument continues, and there is no clear-cut culprit upon whom to lay the blame.

The second factor in physicians' contribution to the scarcity of resources is that, as there is good reason to believe, they tend to overuse the system. Among the several explanations for overtreating is that American health care consumers are litigious, and many doctors fear being sued. Malpractice insurance for physicians today is astronomically expensive, especially in certain specialty areas. In fact, many newly graduating family physicians refuse to deliver babies since obstetrical cases are among the most frequently litigated and insurance is simply too expensive. Instead, the doctors opt to give up delivering babies, forcing more and more people to more expensive medical care providers – namely, obstetricians. The demanding modern consumer has changed forever the relationship between doctor and patient, and doctors know that if they are found to have neglected to do everything possible for a given patient, they are likely to be sued. This is strong motivation for leaving no treatment stone unturned, no matter how far-fetched it might be.

WHAT EFFECT IS THIS HAVING ON YOU?

You may believe that the scarcity of health care resources is not yet affecting you and your health care. The fact is that you may be wholly unaware of the subtle rationing of health care resources that is going on around you at this very moment; you may not know that you have waited in line. If rationing has not affected your health, then it is probably not a bad thing in and of itself. The problem, however, is that you do not know if you were treated equitably within the system.

As doctors, health economists, administrators, and governments continue to talk about the shortage of health care resources, you might wonder just what resources they are talking about.

Obviously, the first resource that comes to mind, largely because it seems to be the crux of the problem, is money. Health care is not the only thing that the United States and Canada have to spend their financial resources on, but sometimes it seems that it takes the biggest chunk. In fact, 11 per cent of the American gross national product (GNP) and about 9.5 per cent of the Canadian GNP is devoted solely to health care. And we do not even have the healthiest populations, when compared with those of other developed countries. Discussions of the money crunch in health care are not always viewed objectively by health professionals. Many of them seem to believe that discussions of money tend to try to place a value on human life and degrade the noble work that they do. While none of us would like to think that the price-tag of a procedure was the main criterion for deciding whether or not we would receive it, budgetary considerations are very important in the bigger picture. If doctors and other health professionals had been more fiscally responsible through the years, perhaps we wouldn't have to examine their ethics in this area at all.

The second area where resources are in short supply is personnel and equipment. Often, the problem is not one of absolute shortfall. In fact, many areas are what have come to be called 'over-doctored.' For example, many urban areas have too many specialists, while rural and remote areas may not have even one resident physician. This is a case of inappropriate distribution, resulting in scarcity of personnel in some regions. The same holds true of equipment. Some cities have so many MRI machines to take three-dimensional pictures of the inside of people's bodies that they are practically using them to diagnose hangnails, whereas patients in some areas must wait months to be scanned.

Money, personnel, beds, equipment, time, energy, and donor organs are all in short supply much of the time. The result is direct problems for individual patients and indirect problems for all of us. If we do not do something about this, our health care concerns promise to grow larger.

HOW CAN DOCTORS BE FAIR?

There ought to be a good way to make good decisions about who should get what, and while various approaches to ensuring the best distribution of scarce resources have been suggested, these are not always applied well in practice.

Here are some of those suggestions:

1. We could give to everyone according to his or her *ability to pay*. Only those who could afford health care would get it; those who could not would simply have to do without. If health care were only a consumer commodity and not something to which everyone is entitled, this would seem like an ethically acceptable way to approach distribution. On the other hand, if health care is perceived as a right, then this approach is immoral. The rich should not be entitled to any more than the poor. One system for those who can pay and a second for those who cannot is what you often hear referred to as the 'two-tiered health care system.' There is a great deal of criticism directed at this approach in both the United States and Canada.

2. Perhaps, instead, we should give to each according to his or her *contributions to society*. This approach would give a bigger piece of the pie to those who have made significant contributions to North American society or who have the potential to do so. The problem here is that a different value is placed on individual human beings, which, according to our human-rights beliefs, is morally unacceptable. But does it go on today? The potential certainly exists. If there is one bed available in the intensive care unit and there are two patients the same age and with equivalent medical conditions who could each benefit from that care, it is difficult for physicians to be completely objective in deciding whether to give the bed to the employed father of three or to the indigent alcoholic from the shelter for the homeless.

3. Another approach would be go give to each *according to his or her age*. In other words, we could decide that younger people

are entitled to greater consideration (on the other hand, if we venerated the elderly, as is done in some other cultures, we might decide the opposite). This ageism, or discrimination on the basis of age, is already occurring. According to one medical researcher who studied patients with kidney disease in both the United States and Canada, there is age discrimination in the allocation of resources for their care (McCann 1993). After studying kidney-failure patients over a three-year period in Alberta and a two-year period in Minnesota, he found that, while 80–100 per cent of those patients aged fourteen to forty-five were accepted into dialysis programs, by the time patients reached age seventy-five the acceptance rate fell to 8 per cent in Alberta and 13 per cent in Minnesota. As for their chances of receiving a kidney transplant, dialysis patients under age forty-four years were transplanted 60–100 per cent of the time and, of those over age seventy-five, none was transplanted in the U.S. part of the study, and only 2 per cent were in the Canadian part. The report of the study did not indicate if any other factors, such as the presence of other diseases, might have accounted for some of this difference.

4. It would seem fair that a person should receive medical care *according to his or her need*. While this approach may seem morally acceptable, the problem is that the medical profession has been singularly unable to determine what exactly it is that people need, short of everything that medical science has to offer. Most doctors believe that each of their patients should have the best available care. Few patients would disagree. But few of us as individuals, doctors included, consider that failure to consider how much is available overall can affect others. It has fallen to governments to try to determine what constitutes good, basic health care.

5. Another approach that seems to some people to be fair is to give to a person *according to his or her place in line*. In other words, first come, first served. While this has its obvious advantages in terms of justice, it would likely result in distribution of health care resources that had no basis at all in medical necessity, a factor which everyone seems to think has at

least some merit. For example, if two people were admitted through the emergency room at the same time and both needed the one available bed in the coronary-care unit, the one who came through the door first should get the bed, based on this approach to resource allocation, even if the second patient is more likely to benefit that the first from coronary care. If this approach were adopted, often sicker people would have to stand in line behind those who are less sick, waiting their turn.

6. In many situations, it would probably be fairer to give the resources based on some kind of *lottery*. If there are two hearts available for transplant tonight and there are three patients who have compatible blood and who could all benefit, leave out their age, sex, socio-economic status, ability to pay, and all the rest of it, and draw the recipient's name out of a hat. In the final analysis, since medical practitioners seem to have such difficulty saying 'no' for a variety of reasons, this might be the easiest approach. The easiest, however, is not always the fairest. It is always easier to make decisions about who should not receive medical care when you are making those decisions from afar. If you are an administrator or a politician, or even a member of the general public who has no direct involvement in a particular case, it is easy to say no. As one writer put it: 'It is easier to say no to invisible people; it is much harder to say no to a person who has a face, a family and a name' (Rooks 1990, 43).

A SPECIAL PROBLEM: SELF-INFLICTED MEDICAL NEEDS

Should people who contribute to their own health problems have equal access to health care resources, whether basic or extended? Should people who smoke have equal access to heart surgery or treatment for lung cancer? Should people who drink too much be eligible on an equal basis with others for liver transplantation? Should people who fail to take any responsibility for their own health have the same rights as those who are more careful? While stopping some of these behaviours that affect health adversely may be difficult, experience indicates that it is not impossible, and starting them in the first place is a matter of choice.

These are difficult questions, and have yet to be answered by the gatekeepers of our health care systems. What has become increasingly popular is the notion that, in today's information society, few health care consumers have any excuse for not knowing how to take care of their health, and therefore have a duty to keep as healthy as possible.

We also need to be realistic about what modern medicine can do for us. Whether we like it or not, we will all die some day, and most of us will suffer from some degree of debilitation as we age. Doctors are as guilty as anyone for generating unrealistic expectations in their patients, and you need to be aware of this. Doctors do not like to lose patients and will often do anything possible to avoid this.

WHO SHOULD BE MAKING THE DECISIONS?

Doctors see themselves as being at the interface between their patients and the system. In this way, they are often the gatekeepers when it comes to use of health care resources. The question is: should they be the gatekeepers? Not even doctors can agree about this one.

Some doctors feel very strongly that they do not want to be the ones to make those global decisions. They want to be left to give medical care to their own patients and to make decisions in the context of the individual doctor–patient encounter. On the other hand, other doctors believe that they should play an even bigger role. In 1991, one doctor wrote: 'it is my belief that we, as physicians, must take increased responsibility for resource allocation. This means withholding diagnostic procedures from some patients, and therapeutic interventions from others' (Smith 1991, vi).

We can only hope that the physicians who are making these decisions have a sound basis in ethical decision making and are equal to the task. We're not so sure that this is a given.

WHAT YOU CAN DO

Most of the allocation decisions that will have to be made in the future in our health care systems are likely to be less individual ones and more broad, society-based ones about what should be provided to whom and how. In other words, we will see the development of general principles and societal policies, much of the impetus for which is coming from governments. It would be a great comfort to every educated health care consumer to have a say in what decisions are going to be made. To ensure that you are informed about the decision-making process, you can do the following:

- Take advantage of any available opportunity to listen to what is being said and to give your opinion on health policy issues. If a government-sponsored forum on health care comes to your town, attend or, at the very least, follow the story in the media.
- Whenever there is an election in your community – municipal, state/provincial, or federal – try to find out the various candidates' views on health care reform. Your vote can be a very powerful voice when it comes to these changes.
- If you are involved in any health-related non-profit organization, encourage it to present a belief statement to local government officials.
- If you feel strongly about an issue related to the fair allocation of health care resources, gather as much information as you can from city and university libraries, media morgues, and related organizations, and begin your own lobby.

8

Strange Bedfellows: Doctors and Drug Manufacturers

Dr Goode had just returned from delivering a baby during the middle of his busy office hours. As he stepped off the elevator, he sighed, hoping that the patients were not stacked up in the waiting-room. He hoped that his receptionist had been diligent enough to reschedule some, and send others off to see one of his partners. Finding only three people waiting to see him, his faith in his receptionist was once again restored. One, however, was not a patient but a 'drug rep' (also known as a 'detail man' in earlier days) from a pharmaceutical company.

After he had seen the remaining patients, Dr Goode let the drug salesperson into his office. They knew each other from many such encounters in the past. The salesperson extended her hand to Dr Goode. Dr Goode shook it.

'Thanks so much for seeing me today, Dr Goode.'

She placed her large sample case on the floor beside her chair and removed a large package, which she placed on the desk. 'I have some information and samples of one of our newest drugs. We're getting a lot of good feedback from the docs who have already started using it.'

Dr Goode took the brochure which the sales rep offered to him. 'I haven't had much use for this yet,' he said.

'That's why I'm here today. We're hoping that you will take part in some research on this drug.'

'What kind of research? Hasn't it already been approved for use?'

'Of course.' The woman waved her hand dismissively. 'But, as you know, we are always testing these drugs for effect, and for side-effects. We are putting specially equipped computers in doctors' offices to keep track of the patients. After you have placed ten patients on this drug and entered the data, your part in the study will be over. Of course, you will be able to keep the computer at that time. We won't have any use for it.'

Dr Goode thought about the patient whose baby he had delivered earlier and nodded absently. The sales rep took that to be a consent and began to get up, while telling him when they were likely to arrive with the computer.

When she left, Dr Goode began to think about what had just happened and decided that perhaps he didn't want to take part in the study after all. The computer seemed like an enticement to prescribe a certain kind of drug, and he didn't like that. He liked to make his decisions based on what he felt the patient needed, without pressure from a drug company. He made a note to call the territory manager in the morning.

Drug manufacturers are arguably the single most important private industry associated with health care today. There are some very specific reasons for this conclusion:

- Their products are directly consumed by hundreds of millions of patients every day. You are likely one of them.
- The most sophisticated of these products are available to patients only because doctors prescribe them.
- Drug companies spend millions of dollars every year promoting their products to physicians.
- Drug companies spend millions of dollars every year supporting medical research.
- Countless doctors attend educational seminars that are supported in one way or another by funds from drug manufacturers.

And, if you think that doctors are not at all influenced by these manufacturers and their skilful marketing tactics, you are not alone. Doctors generally think that too. The influence may be very subtle, but it can be there.

THE INFLUENCES OF PHARMACEUTICALS PRODUCERS ON DOCTORS

Ask a doctor if he or she is influenced by drug-company tactics to prescribe certain drugs and that doctor will likely respond with an emphatic 'no.' The problem seems to be that doctors do not even know that they are being influenced.

For many years, all you had to do was walk through a large teaching hospital to see which drug reps had been around recently. The 'house staff' – interns, residents, and medical students – looked like walking advertisements for drug companies. They had pocket protectors that sported drug-company logos, pens with company names, notepads and even prescription pads with particular drugs advertised. Then a walk into a doctor's office would show you drug-company mugs, paperweights, and posters. A glimpse of an off-duty doctor might show you ball caps, tee-shirts, umbrellas, carry-bags, and just about anything else that could be emblazoned with advertising. Surely all this advertising must exert *some* influence. Otherwise, why do drug companies do it?

In a study conducted at Case Western Reserve University in Cleveland, researchers wanted to see if indeed these interactions with drug companies actually influenced the prescribing behaviour of doctors. They interviewed physicians who had asked to have specific, brand-name drugs added to the hospital pharmacy's regular list of inventory. During the interviews, these doctors were unaware of the objective of the study, so this could not influence their answers. What the research found was that doctors requesting specific drugs were about four times more likely than were doctors in a control group who had not requested drugs by name to have met with the specific drug-company representative as they were to have met with reps from other companies. They also found that the requesting doctors were two and a half times more likely to have accepted funds from the specific drug company. These funds were to support their attendance at meetings, to give a presentation, or to do research of one kind or another (Gullens 1992). It seems, then that the enormous amount of money allotted every year by drug companies for promoting their products to physicians is well spent.

THE COST OF DRUG PROMOTION

Just how much money is spent by drug manufacturers on promotion to doctors? According to a study conducted by a special panel for the Canadian Public Health Association, drug companies spend about 25 per cent of their annual sales, or $10,000 annually per physician, on marketing and promotion. This covers a wide variety of promotional activities:

- direct marketing through sending brochures to doctors' offices
- visits to doctors' offices by drug salespeople
- support of continuing medical education activities
- provision of samples to doctors
- coverage of travel expenses for doctors to attend drug company–sponsored activities
- rental of booths in exhibition areas at medical meetings
- advertisements in medical journals and magazines
- 'ghost-written' articles in what doctors call 'throw-away' medical journals that promote a drug indirectly – articles by professional medical writers appearing under doctors' names and published by magazines that are produced by drug companies

And there are other, more innovative, strategies used by some pharmaceutical manufacturers.

Clearly, drug companies have a lot to gain by promoting their wares to doctors. In the end, though, is this really a problem for patients? As we shall see next, there certainly can be problems for patients and their rights if doctors don't behave themselves.

THE POST-MARKETING STUDY AND YOU

Most members of the general public, and even some newly graduated doctors, are unaware of something called 'a post-marketing study' of a drug sponsored wholly by the company that manufactures it. Before we look at the problems such studies represent for both doctors and patients, let us examine what they are.

In both Canada and the United States, a very elaborate bureaucratic and scientific system is in place for the testing and approval of new drugs before they can enter the marketplace and be prescribed by doctors. In Canada, the Health Protection Branch (HPB) is the agency responsible, and in the United States it is the Food and Drug Administration (FDA). The process is complex, and can take a very long time. From a patient's point of view, that should be a good thing. The more testing that is done, the less likelihood there will be for surprises when the drug is widely available. On the down side, lengthy testing sometimes causes difficulties for people awaiting a specific drug that is already available in other parts of the world. The bottom line is that, although no guarantees of either safety or efficacy are made, drugs are well tested before they reach consumers.

Drug companies, however, to their credit, do not leave it at that. They continually test their drugs, and ask doctors to observe the patients they have placed on these drugs. As commendable as this may be in theory, it may not always appear that way to either the doctors or the patients involved. The problems are not related to the fact that these studies are being done, but to *how* they are being done.

Here's what happens. A letter arrives at the doctor's office, more often than you can imagine, phrased something like this:

Dear Doctor:
XXXX drug has been approved for the treatment of XXX. It promises to bring the power ...

We are therefore inviting a select group of general practitioners to study the potential impact of XXXX on their practices ...

To this end I would like to invite you to participate ...

The attachments to the inviting letter indicate that there will be a first meeting where a doctor of some local repute will make a presentation on his or her personal experience with the drug. This will include a scientific review of the drug. The second phase of the study is a 'clinical experience' where the doctors will study the effects of the drug on patients in their own practices. Then there will be a meeting to evaluate the process after which each participant will receive an honorarium of $400. There are no specifics about either the nature of the 'clinical experience' or the location of the evaluation meeting (possibly the Bahamas?).

While this might seem innocuous enough and surely inviting for the doctor, most doctors themselves have come to the conclusion that they are entering shaky ethical territory when they become involved in these projects that result in personal gain for them. Doctors need to be concerned about whether their clinical judgment is being unduly influenced by taking part and they need to be particularly careful about how they gain patient consent for participation, because the patient does, indeed, need to be able to make an informed decision about participation.

One of the 'perks' of these studies is that the drug under examination is often supplied to the patient free-of-charge for the duration of the study. After the study is over, the patient will have to begin paying for it. Some doctors have expressed concern that if a drug has a good effect on a patient, the doctor is unlikely to change it and newer preparations tend to be much more costly than the old stand-bys. But that is not the most serious problem for the patient.

The most serious breach of ethics by doctors engaged in these studies is the difficulty that they sometimes have in gaining patient participation without making the patient feel coerced into it. It isn't that the doctor does this intentionally, but the patient can feel pressured anyway. For example, if you were an older adult on a fixed income and someone offered you your needed drugs free, would you not feel 'pressured' to participate? Truly informed consent is almost impossible to guarantee in these cases. As well, it is possible for the 'perks,' whether they are money, equipment, or even trips, to affect a doctor's objectivity. Doctors are, after all, as we have said before, only human. This is one of the main criticisms of these studies from the patient's point of view.

Organized medicine in North America is, however, trying to do something about this situation.

NEW GUIDELINES FOR DOCTORS

The primary objective of professional interactions between physicians and the pharmaceutical industry should be the advancement of the health of Canadians rather than the private good of either physicians or industry.

This is the first of the general principles in the Canadian Medical Association's recent (1994) guidelines for physicians and the pharmaceutical industry. While it is widely accepted that doctors should place the patient above all else, the notion of a medical association presuming to make such proclamations for the pharmaceutical industry borders on the ludicrous. Clearly, they are ignoring the free-market system within which these companies function and flourish. The fact is that drug companies are in business to make money. In so doing, their approach might be to attempt to do good and to do no harm, as the physician does, but for them to ignore their profit-making function would be irresponsible to both their investors and their employees. So, what we are left with is the fact that we have to place a good deal of responsibility for maintaining the ethical purity of these encounters on the shoulders of doctors. Are they up to it?

Recent correspondence in the *Canadian Medical Association Journal* indicates quite clearly that doctors are insulted by the notion that their association would imply that they are involved in shady dealings with drug companies. In one letter to the editor, the doctor-author had this to say:

Physicians and the innovative pharmaceutical industry by and large have ethical and appropriate conduct. Before we become too critical of the industry we should reflect on the advances made in therapeutics over the past 15 years, which, through providing physicians with tools to treat patients more efficiently and effectively, have far surpassed all other advances in health care. (Arkinstall 1993, 485)

Another said this of the guidelines:

Moses came up with some very famous and noble guidelines, and we all know how religiously they are being followed today ... Let's catch the bad apples and punish them appropriately and not waste our time, effort and money in restating the obvious ad nauseam. (Jablonsky 1993, 486)

Doctors are become increasingly wary of drug companies and their approaches to research and marketing and the relationship between the two. One of the main difficulties with this apprehension is that it is becoming harder to differentiate between the truly useful, ethical study and the questionable one. In addition, some doctors say that they are even shying away from medications that have recently been presented to them by sales representatives for fear of being accused of being influenced in their treatment decisions by drug companies. The best interests of the patient ought to guide the medical decision.

WHAT YOU CAN DO

As a patient, how can you feel comfortable that you are being given optimum treatment when faced with a post-marketing surveillance study? Obviously, one approach would simply be to refuse such participation. However, that is not necessarily in your best interests. The drug that is being studied might very well be the best drug for you. Furthermore, if all patients refused, we would lose a source of information that could prove useful in the future.

Here are some suggestions for the circumstances under which you might feel comfortable participating in such a study:

- The doctor has explained the alternative treatments to you.
- The doctor has already made a decision about your treatment and presented it to you before mentioning any drug study.
- You feel no pressure to take part simply because the drugs will be provided free of charge.
- The doctor has explained what information he or she will have to provide about you for the researchers.
- The doctor has explained how your medical information will be kept confidential or anonymous.

If you do feel comfortable about all of the above items, you are probably in a good position to give informed consent. This is very much like giving consent for other medical procedures, as we discussed earlier. Read the form before you sign it and ask your doctor to keep you informed about how the study is going and what they ultimately discover about the drug.

These circumstances are not unlike those we discussed earlier regarding your right to give informed consent. In fact, the notion of informed consent is one of the issues at the heart of the drug company–physician problems.

If you look around you doctor's office and see every imaginable type of paraphernalia emblazoned with drug-company logos, you might want to ask your doctor what he or she had to do to get them. It would be worth noting the reaction to the question.

PART II

HIGH-TECH MEDICAL ETHICS:
ISSUES FOR SOME

The next five chapters will take you inside some important areas of what is high-technology medicine today and help you to see the kinds of ethical problems that face doctors and other health professionals. Not everyone will be directly affected in life by this kind of medical service, but the ethical decisions that have an impact on resources or speak directly to some of the societal moral concerns have implications for everyone.

This discussion of technological approaches to health care is not exhaustive, but it is designed to give you, the health care consumer, a better idea of what issues are being grappled with today.

9

High-Tech Medicine:
Who Needs It?

Dr Ursula Rebecca Smart, MD, FACS, FRCS(C), walked into her office at midnight and flopped herself into the chair facing her desk. She was exhausted. She looked at the pile of charts on her desk, the unopened mail, the piece she had been reading at five-thirty when this evening's marathon had begun.

The Director of Intensive Care Services at a large, urban teaching hospital, she sometimes found herself yearning for those days before she had chosen her specialty. She had spent two years as a family doctor who could recognize her patients on the street and speak to all the kids by name. Then, when her reverie ended, she would realize that she was exactly where she wanted to be. The excitement and fast pace of the latest in high-tech medicine were but a few steps away, outside her office door. And that, together with the rush she got every time she realized that they had saved another life, was what she thrived on. It was only in the moments after unsuccessful attempts to save a life that she wondered why she did it.

She leaned towards the desk and picked up the notes on the top of the pile of charts. It was the case for tomorrow morning's grand rounds. Her resident would present the details of the patient, and Dr Smart would conduct the discussion. Those in attendance would learn something.

The name on the top sheet was 'Alvarez, Maria.' Below this it read, 'Female, thirty-five years old, motor vehicle accident.' As she read down the sheet, Dr Smart reviewed X-ray reports, blood chemistry reports, heart monitor strip reports, blood gas figures, and on and on. She realized that she had never known this patient as much more than the sum total of her recorded medical data. Maria had been unconscious since that night two weeks ago when the medics had flown through the doors of the emergency room, holding her intravenous bag overhead and shouting a litany of problems to the nurses: possible head injury, possible internal injuries, fractured tibia and fibula (leg bones), fractured pelvis, fractured ribs, collapsed lung. Maria had been almost dead, but they had managed to save her. They had done everything they could during those two weeks. She had undergone several major surgical procedures and all manner of modern diagnostic tests. She had received intensive nursing care and intensive care from the physiotherapists. She had died only half an hour ago. If only there had been something more they could have done.

Just then, Dr Smart heard a faint knock on her office door. An older woman and a younger man walked in.

'Dr Smart?' the older woman began tentatively. Dr Smart nodded.

'Dr Smart, I am Maria Alvarez's mother, and this is her husband. We have been talking with your residents during the past week and we are grateful for what you have done. Maria was a very strong and happy woman, but she would not have wanted to live with so many problems. Thank you for stopping it all tonight.' They turned and left.

Dr Smart watched them leave and looked down at the pages in front of her. 'Alvarez, Maria. I would have liked to talk to you.' She took off her lab coat and went home.

There is a story in modern medicine that has been told over and over again. Not unlike an urban folktale, the story has a basis in fact, although those facts have likely been embellished in the telling. None the less, the story has an important lesson for physicians and patients alike.

The story begins in the intensive care unit of a large, urban teaching hospital. The intensive care unit is, arguably, the area in the delivery of modern health care where the highest level of technology available for actual care meets the patients. The senior resident had arrived on the unit to make his own early-morning rounds. As he was perusing the strips indicating his patient's heart rhythm and the laboratory reports, he noticed that the cardiac-monitor screen at the desk did not seem to be working properly. The rhythm had changed dramatically. He immediately picked up the telephone and called the biomedical engineering department.

'This is Dr Brown in the ICU,' he began. 'One of our monitors is malfunctioning and we need someone up here stat to fix it. The lives of these patients depend on this equipment, you know.' The technician said he would be there on the double.

When the technician arrived a mere three minutes later, he began the laborious task of uncovering the origin of the malfunction. He started at the nursing station where the remote monitor was located and followed the connections back to the patient's bedside. He inspected the wall receptacle and continued back to where the machine was actually attached to the patient. He finally uncovered the problem for the doctor. The patient was dead.

Haven't figured out the moral of the story yet? It seems that the scientifically sophisticated gadgets available to modern medicine today have changed the art of medicine. That art relies on the doctor's actual hands-on approach and his or her use of intuition. While this may seem like an exaggeration, it is really not too far from the cold reality of high-level technology in North American hospitals of the 1990s.

High-tech medicine encompasses those diagnostic and therapeutic approaches that rely on the latest in medical and pharmaceutical advances. These advances are often available only in urban referral centres, require medical practitioners with specialized training, and are often extraordinarily expensive. Some of these technological marvels include:

• Organ and tissue transplantation (including human-to-human and animal-to-human and the use of fetal tissue);

- Artificial organs (hearts, kidneys, and, the latest, livers);
- Artificial ventilation (respirators);
- Open-heart surgery;
- Laparoscopic surgery (using tiny fibre-optic scope to do surgery that once required large incisions);
- Imaging machines (diagnostic tools that provide three-dimensional views of the insides of our bodies, unlike old X-rays);
- Fetal surgery (surgical correction of defects discovered in unborn babies while *in utero*);
- Extracorporeal shock-wave lithotripsy (pulverization of kidney stones and gallstones with shock waves) . . .

The list gets longer every day. What is becoming increasingly clear is that medical research directed towards the development and testing of new medical-technological breakthroughs is perhaps the fastest-growing area of scientific investment. This is exciting. But this commercial aspect of medical technology has recently begun to add to the growing concerns about whether we are controlling the technology or the technology is controlling us.

HIGH-TECH'S HISTORICAL DEVELOPMENT

Oliver Wendell Holmes should be well known to every doctor in practice today as an important historical figure in this complex discipline. A nineteenth century American physician-author, Holmes was a professor of anatomy and physiology at Harvard. He was more than a physician-teacher, though, as he was an artist as well as a scientist, writing poetry and fiction in addition to medical papers. In 1872 he wrote: 'Science is a first-rate piece of furniture for a man's upper chamber if he has common sense on the ground floor.' This admonition is still as useful today as it was a hundred years ago, and many would argue that the medical profession, despite its scientific advances, has yet to discover a good dose of Holmes's common sense.

Despite the fact that the practice of medicine dates back some

2,400 years, to the origins of the Hippocratic tradition and beyond, only since the nineteenth century has medicine had any real basis in scientific discovery. The mind-set of modern medical science, however, can be traced back to Francis Bacon in seventeenth-century England. By all accounts, one of his greatest contributions to the world was his development of a new type of inductive reasoning that was applied to scientific thought; this style of reasoning formed the basis for modern scientific inquiry, becoming the method used to conduct modern scientific research. More than this, though, Bacon's new approach to science could be used to exercise control over nature.

It was another two hundred years, though, before the practice of medicine began to really identify itself with science. Until this time, the Hippocratic approach to medicine, which encompassed the philosophy of working with nature to heal the patient, dominated medical thought. Scientists tended to view medicine as an art rather than a science. With the founding of the American Medical Association in 1847, medicine set itself up as a scientific approach to healing, in contrast to other types of healing practised at the time.

Considerable discussion in the medical literature is devoted to the limits of science. What all this discussion tells us is that, first, there is no general agreement among physicians about the place that art, as opposed to science, has in the practice of medicine, and, second, that they are concerned about where medicine as a science is headed. As one writer put it, 'Baconian science, a tool for plundering nature, has impelled physicians to insist on medical treatment, even when it is futile. The Hippocratic tradition of medicine teaches us instead to acknowledge nature's limits' (Jecker 1991, 5). It is these 'natural' limits and their place in medical science that are not clearly understood by either doctors on the verge of new technologies or health care consumers.

There is little doubt in anyone's mind that we are better off today with all our medical marvels than we were at the turn of the century. Physicians did not have the tools to cure disease; they could only treat the symptoms. The problem is that these new-found powers over life and death have left us with a legacy of moral dilemmas that neither doctors nor the public have come even close to solving. Doctors and other health professionals now often revere the scientific approach to health care delivery as if it were some kind of a god itself, with illness and disability a devil. This is illustrated even in the way we pay caregivers in North America.

'Technique-oriented procedures receive greater compensation than do cognitive acts ... the "laying on of hands"' (James and colleagues 1990, 264). In other words, those involved in the 'cutting specialties,' such as neurosurgeons, heart surgeons, and ophthalmologists (eye surgeons), receive higher pay for their work than do those who spend more time thinking and caregiving, such as specialists in internal medicine and family medicine. Psychiatrists and pediatricians tend to be at the lowest end of the pay scale.

Even the nursing contracts that govern salaries of registered nurses across both Canada and the United States put a premium on work in 'technical' areas, such as intensive care, the operating room, and the emergency department. While it is argued that a nurse in the ICU requires specialized training beyond his or her basic nursing education, consider the following comparison: a nurse who works in the ICU on a given shift will have, perhaps, one patient for whom he or she is totally responsible. The areas of responsibility include the use of a variety of machinery, such as artificial ventilators, intravenous infusion pumps, and cardiac monitors, all of which require special post-graduate training, whether on the job or as part of a course. On the same shift, another nurse may be charged with the care of, say, six cancer patients who require less technological care, but who are facing impending death. This nurse may even have to sit with one of these patients to await death on this shift. This nurse requires highly developed communication and counselling skills, in addition to the basic skills of nursing care. Is one of these nurses more valuable than the other? If we use remuneration as the yardstick, evidently the ICU nurse is, as he or she is the one who will receive a premium on the shift rate.

There is little doubt that high-technology care is becoming a major part of our health care delivery system. For example, while intensive care beds typically account for only 5 per cent of hospital bed capacity, they eat up 20 per cent of the total hospital budgets (Technology Subcommittee of the Working Group on Critical Care, 1991). One of the persistent problems with this head-long rush into technology that seems to be beckoning a large proportion of physicians today is that some of this new technology is adopted without very clear knowledge of how well it will work out. Assessing the value of new technological approaches to giving medical care is not an easy task, and it is very expensive. The problem is that some technological marvels later turn out to have severely limited usefulness. Doctors have recently developed this habit of latching on to technology and taking the patient along for the ride. It has been estimated that as many as 80 per cent of all medical approaches have not actually been well evaluated (Rachlis and Kushner 1989).

One example is a procedure called a carotid endarterectomy. This is a surgical procedure that involves scraping deposits off the interior walls of the artery leading to the brain in an attempt to prevent strokes. (The carotid artery is the pulse point in the neck that you often use to check your heart rate during aerobic workouts.) The procedure itself carries with it a risk of stroke or death. While this procedure has been done since the 1960s, there has never been any clear evidence that it is useful. As some people began to doubt its usefulness and worry about its unpleasant effects, a study was begun in 1987, involving patients in both Canada and the United States to evaluate it. This procedure was one of the medical approaches that was studied by the Rand Corporation of Santa Monica, California, when they embarked on an examination of unnecessary medical treatment. When they looked at the results obtained by some 1,300 elderly patients who had undergone the procedure, they found that almost one-third of them hadn't needed it ('Wasted health care dollars,' 1992).

Another study compared both the treatment and its results in heart patients in Canada and the United States. After studying

1,574 American and 657 Canadian patients, all of whom were treated in university or university-affiliated hospitals where all patients had medical insurance coverage, the researchers reported some very interesting results. First, they discovered that American patients were treated much more vigorously, with more surgical procedures and more drug therapy, than were the Canadian patients. Their second finding, however, was that there was virtually no difference in death rates or in the number of heart patients who were likely to suffer another heart attack in spite of the differences in treatment approach (Kucharesky 1992). This called into serious question the reasoning behind subjecting so many people to such invasive and expensive treatment approaches.

On the other hand, we need to acknowledge the fact that some technological marvels have contributed in no small way to more effective and efficient medical care. For example, in years past, any person who required abdominal surgery for any reason had to undergo a major surgical procedure called a laparotomy. It involved a large incision and a relatively lengthy hospital stay. In an increasing number of cases, today's technology allows surgeons to do this surgery through a small scope, a laparoscope, requiring only a tiny incision. In these cases, the patient can often go home the day of the surgery or after a significantly shortened stay. Shorter hospital stays are good for the patient and decrease costs.

There are still concerns for health care consumers when it comes to high-technology medicine. It is easy to be seduced by the high-profile media stories into thinking that there are few, if any, problems with all this progress.

While MRIs, CT scans, lasers, super drugs, and all the other wonders of modern medicine have, at least to some extent, contributed to a better understanding of both human health and disease and care for some people, it has not been achieved without a cost – and not merely a financial one. Indeed, there are specific areas where patients are or should be concerned about the state of modern health care.

THE DISTANCE BETWEEN DOCTORS AND PATIENTS

The first problem that high-tech medicine has had for the patient is that it has *increased the distance between you and your medical caregiver.* It has not only placed a physical barrier between you, as in the case of diagnostic machines, but also contributed to the creation of an intellectual barrier.

Many patients find that doctors no longer have the same interest in hands-on caring, as they reach for their prescription pads and diagnostic requisitions. There was a time when the physician placed his or her ear directly on the patient's chest to listen to the heart beat, and even tasted the patient's sweat and urine. While we are not suggesting that we need to revert to this kind of closeness, it illustrates the increasing distance that is threatening the human side of the practice of medicine. The way modern medical care is delivered fragments the patient into systems, organs, chemicals, and electrical impulses. The person is now the sum of all the tests performed on his or her body.

WHOM CAN YOU BELIEVE?

The second problem stems from the high-profile nature of many of the technological marvels. Media stories are much more likely to relate to so-called breakthroughs than to focus on the more mundane, thus we are bombarded by news of medical discoveries. The problem for the patient, then, is *not knowing whom to believe.*

A recent high-profile controversy that continues to rage relates to the usefulness of mammography. Stories have appeared everywhere, from the local media to national women's magazines, to medical journals, each with a slightly different slant. When a not-quite-forty woman walks into her doctor's office and is confronted with the question of whether or not to have a baseline mammogram, whose guidelines is she to follow? Does she take her own doctor's recommendation at face value? Does she ask for a second opinion? Does she draw her own conclusions from what she has recently read or seen or heard in the media? Does she ask a friend? It seems to be very difficult for a patient to know whom to believe, but, in fact, you may need to rely on information from more than one source.

If you have developed a solid relationship with a family doctor whose knowledge and judgment you respect and who has proven him or herself to be capable of helping you to understand your medical care, and whose values you either share or, at the very least, understand, this is a good place to start gathering your information. Your doctor can help you to interpret what you are seeing and hearing about your own medical problem, and might even suggest that you talk to another physician. One approach that you should be wary of, though, is relying primarily on information from a friend who has had the same problem. This person may overidentify with the situation so much that he or she may overlook the fact that *you* are the patient in question.

KNOWING WHEN TO STOP

Another doctor-related problem in high-tech medicine is *the physician who does not know when to stop*. This doctor is generally viewed by colleagues as lacking in confidence about his or her own medical capabilities. Whether this attitude about death as the enemy is an innate fear in people who choose medicine as a career or is ingrained by medical schools has never been sorted out. It is, however, a growing problem among the younger physicians of today.

This problem stems from advances in modern medicine. Years ago, even if the doctor didn't want to stop treating a patient, his or her resources were severely limited by the state of available medical approaches. The doctor was forced into a decision to stop treating because of a lack of alternatives. Today, there is such an array of possibilities that it may take a very long time for all of them to be exhausted. Other factors today, however, can contribute to a decision to stop treating. One of these is lack of accessibility. If the medical approach that is the next step for your problem is inaccessible to you because of such factors as geographic distance, this will play a part in the treatment decision. Another of these factors may be cost. Someone has to pay for medical treatment, and sometimes the cost, coupled with the medical prognosis, contributes to the decision to stop treating.

TECHNOLOGY, FREE ENTERPRISE, AND DOCTORS

Another issue that becomes problematic for the patient is *the growing health care technology business within a free-enterprise system, and its relationship with doctors.* If a company develops a piece of equipment, it markets it aggressively. When a physician or a hospital purchases this particular piece of expensive medical equipment, it is necessary for that physician or hospital to pay for it. The way to pay for it is to use it so that the money is recouped from the government, the patient, or a private insurance company.

If a group of physicians owns their own laboratories, patients can never be certain that there is no conflict of interest. As convenient as it may be for patients to have one-stop shopping, so to speak, patients have to be wary of overuse of lab testing in these instances. A doctor who makes a profit from an on-site laboratory might be guilty of overuse of blood testing. This is certainly not true in all cases, but it might be helpful to know if the service is simply a welcome convenience for the patient or a money-making venture for the doctor. If you are concerned, ask. Again, if you have developed a good relationship with a doctor, the discussion might be a very informative one. If you are just beginning your association with a doctor, keep track of the blood tests you are having. If it appears to you that there is a significant increase, some investigation by you is warranted. A doctor should be able to give you a clear, rational explanation for each test that is ordered.

SO MANY HEALTH FIELDS

Finally, and perhaps the most obviously bewildering for patients, as health care technology increases, *there has been a baffling increase in the number of different allied health fields.* What the patient may not know is that each group is jockeying for position in the race for a piece of the health care pie. A discipline that can claim a new procedure for itself enhances its own position and wins the fee for that service. The problem for the patient is the baffling number of people involved in the treatment equation, all of whom have specific specialty areas, none of which is really well known to the average consumer.

Prior to the use of ultrasound technology, for example, there was no need for ultrasound technologists. Prior to the introduction of open-heart surgery and dialysis, there were no perfusionists. If you are admitted to the hospital today, you will be faced with an enormous number of caregivers, many of whom will deliver a type of 'care' that may be a mystery to you. Today, alongside the traditional health occupations of medicine and nursing are some 700 specialty, subspecialty, and sub-subspecialty fields within health care delivery. Many of these are new, and the list is growing. As we have already discussed, the growth in numbers of people who will care for you increases the risk of breach of confidentiality. In addition, it fragments the care you receive and makes you feel, not like a person, but like a collection of molecules, chemicals, organs, and body systems. This is another factor that has contributed to the dehumanization of medical care.

On the other hand, this degree of specialization means that the person who is doing a procedure on you does that kind of work all day long, with the result that the quality of the service delivered is likely to be higher.

THE MODERN DILEMMA

Some critics have said that, if health care facilities have the latest in medical technological equipment, they are more likely to attract and keep top-notch physicians. In some communities, having such equipment is what might help to attract any physician at all. In many cases, this view is accurate. While the priority given to high-tech equipment may have some important positive consequences for some patients, it is becoming increasingly clear that not all the results are quite so beneficial. These misplaced priorities are amply illustrated by a number of similar incidences across the continent. One such instance was related in a recent story in *Consumer Reports*: 'During the 1980's, while American hospitals were falling all over themselves to add costly, high-tech neonatal intensive care units, the number of mothers unable to get basic prenatal care climbed, as did the incidence of premature births' ('Wasted Health Care Dollars ...' 1992, 447).

If there is one single issue that future medical historians might pinpoint as the heart of twentieth-century ethical problems in medicine, it will probably be the fact that medical science has developed at a far faster rate than our ability to deal with the new problems presented by these recently acquired powers over life and death. As modern medicine has increased the quantity of life (almost thirty extra years since the beginning of the century), it has been almost totally unable to come to terms with the quality-of-life issues that have arisen as a consequence.

There has been an increasing concern in the industrialized world for the development of improved assessment processes for new medical technologies. It seems that this is a growth area for business. Both the United States and Canada have government-related offices for the assessment of new medical technologies: the Office of Technology Assessment in the United States, and the Canadian Coordinating Office for Health Technology Assessment. The term 'health technology assessment' means all of the methods necessary for examining new developments in procedures, equipment, and drugs. This examination includes looking at their costs, safety, how well they work, the ethics of their use, and what impact they will have on the quality of life (Huston 1992).

With input from physicians, allied health professionals, administrators, government officials, ethicists, sociologists, and eventually the general public, perhaps there will, indeed, be some progress in developing solutions to these perplexing dilemmas.

As one nursing writer has suggested, if, as the saying goes, politics is too important to leave up to the politicians, then 'the rapid development of advanced technology is too serious to leave up to health personnel' (Quivey 1990, 344).

WHAT YOU CAN DO

We have already alluded to some of the things you can do to play your part in determining if high-technology medical procedures are for you. Here is a summary:

- Be aware of what is being reported in the media about medical marvels. When you are unsure of how to interpret information about those that may have implications for you or your family, talk to you doctor about them.
- Avoid demanding medical procedures. Find out what they involve, how much they cost, whether they might be appropriate for you, and if you would have access to them.
- When you find yourself under the care of a technician or other health care worker whose role you don't understand, ask. The technician who does your ultrasound, for example, would probably be more than happy to talk a little about his or her line of work. If you come into contact with enough of these people, you begin to get a better picture of how modern medical care is delivered.

10

Inside the Intensive Care Unit

Perhaps the modern intensive care unit, especially the one in the university-affiliated, urban hospital, was on American physician-author Samuel Shem's mind when he was preparing what he called the 'Laws of the House of God,' for his irreverent novel *The House of God.* The thirteenth, and last, law is worth remembering: '*The delivery of medical care is to do as much of nothing as possible.*'

While not many people would agree with this as a general principle, some of the approaches taken in the modern intensive care unit seem to many to be just this: a great deal of busy futility. In these days of tempting new medical technology coupled with economic constraints, the ethical problems that emerge from intensive care units seem almost limitless. Here is a sampling of the unanswered questions:

- Who should be treated in intensive care units?
- What kinds of problems should be treated?
- How long should an individual patient be treated?
- Should medical doctors have the right to experiment on gravely ill patients?
- Should medical students use gravely ill patients to practise on?
- How is it decided when to stop the treatment?

Before we examine how these questions are handled in modern

hospitals, let us first take a trip into an intensive care unit to see what happens.

LIFE IN AN ICU

'The capabilities of modern intensive care have no inherent limits' (Cohen 1986, 40). That about sums up what faces you when you pass through the doors of the modern ICU. You face a world where almost anything is theoretically possible, where medical technology stretches itself to its outermost limits, and where few moral dilemmas have been solved to the satisfaction of outsiders.

We begin the tour. The first thing you should notice about the intensive care unit is that it has imposing, visually impenetrable doors. They are supposed to be just that – uninviting. People who work behind those doors do not want you strolling through their corridor, and if you have a friend or relative inside whom you would like to visit, you better be on their 'A' list or you will be shown the other side of the doors very quickly.

Take note of the visiting hours that are usually posted on the door. If you are a close family member, you will likely be permitted to visit for five minutes once an hour. Once that five minutes has been used up, the patient will not be allowed any more visitors until the next hour. While other areas of the hospital might be a bit lax about their enforcement of the visiting-hours policy, this unit will not. Should you overstay your welcome, an assertive nurse will remind you of the posted rules and show you out. And don't bring flowers. They are, at their most innocuous, regarded as unwelcome clutter that interferes with the efficiency of the unit; at their worst, they are a hazard.

Once inside the unit, you will notice a distinctive humming noise in the background, punctuated every so often by beeps that are reminiscent of your microwave and your cellular telephone. Rhythmic whooshing noises provide a restful counterpoint to the cacophony of mechanical sounds and urgent voices. Everyone in a busy ICU seems to have a more important job than you do. Everyone here takes his or her job very seriously, and most are very good at it.

If you peek through the glass into a patient cubicle, you may see a pathetic white-covered lump on a bed with lines and tubes running every which way. There are tubes, wires, and machines to assist with almost every known bodily function. A ventilator breathes for the patient; an intravenous pump ensures the accurate delivery of a solution and likely drugs into the bloodstream; a urine drainage bag attached to a bladder catheter collects urine; a cardiac monitor shows a picture of the electrical conduction in the heart; and, depending upon what specific problems the patient has, other assorted pieces of equipment may be in use.

If you look carefully at the nurses in the ICU, you will notice that they tend to be neither the youngest ones in the hospital (they don't have the experience) nor the oldest (many older nurses find the work stressful). All are paid a higher rate than those in non-special units.

Another thing that you may notice in this big-city hospital ICU is that there are few, if any, empty beds. Since most of the people who require intensive care develop this need urgently, you may wonder what would happen if another patient came to the emergency room and needed an ICU bed. You will not be the only one wondering. The doctor in the emergency room is probably thinking the same thing as he or she deals with the casualties of a major car accident.

If a patient's condition deteriorates while we are on our tour, the team will spring into action immediately. No other nursing unit in the hospital has such an abundance of emergency equipment at close hand, and nowhere else are the nurses and doctors as adept at using it (excluding, of course, the emergency department and operating or recovery rooms, which themselves are also special units).

Generally, intensive care units scare the hell out of the average person, and perhaps this is just as well. There is nothing like a good scare to keep you on your toes and alert to the slightest deviation from the norm, if you know what the norm is! If you were to receive a telephone call tonight that someone you loved dearly had been admitted to the hospital, you would likely be considerably more fearful if that person is being cared for in an ICU. Admission to the ICU means a much more serious illness. That fear manifests itself as helplessness, which leads to the public leaving many of the thorny decisions about medical care under these circumstances to medical personnel.

Many of us know about hospital intensive care units only from our exposure to the television version, where fast-moving, quick-thinking fictitious doctors and nurses minister to the needs of deathly ill fictitious patients with unpronounceable illnesses. Occasionally, a difficult ethical dilemma surfaces as part of the plot, but it is usually overshadowed by the drama, leaving many of the dilemmas shrouded in mystery until we are faced with them in reality.

A UNIT FULL OF QUESTIONS

In order to truly understand the emotional and medical side of the ICU, you need to look beyond the noises and equipment, at the people who occupy the beds. These people, rather than their life-sustaining paraphernalia, are at the heart of the ethical dilemmas that are solved case by case.

Dr Smart met her senior resident at the door of the medical intensive care unit.

'Ready for rounds this morning, Doctor?' she said greeting him. He nodded and pulled the first chart from the rack pushed by the nurse, as they were joined by a junior resident and an intern.

The first patient, Mrs Singh, was a seventy-six-year-old with a long history of severe diabetes resulting in the shut-down of her kidneys. While her kidney function had been slowly worsening, she had been found unconscious by her daughter. On admission to the emergency department, she was in a coma that had developed from her failed kidneys, and her daughter had been told that her mother would die without immediate dialysis. Kidney dialysis machines are sometimes referred to as 'artificial kidneys' because they function to remove toxins from the bloodstream, just as the kidneys do when they are working properly.

We cannot live without our kidney function, and only dialysis several times a week, or a kidney transplant, will save our lives.

As they milled around the bedside, Dr Smart looked over the controls of the dialysis machine and examined Mrs Singh's arm, where the blood tube removed her toxic blood to be cleansed by the machine and returned to her body. The resident noted that Mrs Singh had regained consciousness and that the every-second-day dialysis procedure was effective.

The second patient, Mr Hopkins, was a forty-year-old who had suffered a massive heart attack. His heart has already stopped twice, and cardiopulmonary resuscitation adeptly applied by the ICU staff had saved him. After a course of drug therapy, he was now sitting up in bed, complaining to the nurses about their no-smoking policy and telling everyone that he would do just about anything for a drink of Scotch.

'Mr Hopkins,' the nurse said, 'you know what we've been telling you about your heart condition. Smoking is not permitted in the ICU, and this will be a good chance for you to give up the habit.'

'Lady,' he said, wiping his nose with the back of his hand, 'I been smokin' for thirty years and I ain't likely to stop now, heart attack or no heart attack.'

One of the young doctors winced. Dr Smart examined her patient, and they moved on.

Although the usual stay in the ICU is only about a week, the next patient had already been in the unit for over a month. The victim of a car accident, Mr Johnson was a fifty-year-old who had suffered a major head injury from which the neurosurgeons have said that the likelihood of complete recovery is very small. He was on a ventilator and, despite attempts to wean him off it so that he could breathe on his own, had not been able to breathe independently. The doctors reviewed the latest blood reports and the nurses' notes, wrote new orders, and placed his chart back on the rack.

Just as the little group was rounding the corner of the unit, heading towards the next bed, all of their pagers started bleeping at once, and two nurses rushed by with the 'crash' cart.

'Mr Watson just arrested,' yelled one of the nurses as she flew by. They all ran towards the centre of the drama.

This thirty-year-old man had fallen from the roof of a building while working on it, and he had just suffered cardiac arrest – in other words, his heart had stopped. The flurry of activity was another attempt by the staff to resuscitate him, and their efforts were futile. When Dr Smart realized that the attempt had failed, she looked up at the clock and noted the time of death. After she walked away from the bedside, the senior resident looked at the intern.

'You want some intubation practice?' Since the intern in question had never before done this procedure – passing a breathing tube down into the lungs of a real patient – he eagerly agreed.

Some of the ethical questions presented by these patients' cases may be obvious; others are more subtle. These stories, although they are fictitious, are nevertheless examples of real situations that occur frequently in ICUs. Let us look at some of the dilemmas presented and how doctors deal with them in reality.

First is the question of who should be treated. Is anyone ever too old for these high-tech, expensive technological approaches? Sometimes there is a valid medical reason why an elderly person might not benefit from specific approaches. Indeed, there are also some who believe that older people should move aside to make way for younger people to benefit from up-to-date high-tech medicine. On the other hand, there are those who will never use age as a criterion for stopping treatment. The way this question is handled varies considerably from one location to another. We have heard it said by a member of a transplant team, for example, that the upper limit of age for recipients rises as the head of the department gets older. While this may be a less than objective way of dealing with a serious question, it illustrates the lack of firm foundation for these kind of decisions.

The next question is even more difficult: what kinds of problems should be treated? If a person is suffering from a partially self-inflicted disease and has a lifestyle that continues to contribute to ill health, should that person, who fails to take responsibility for his or her own health, have the same right of access as all others to high-tech medical approaches? For some health professionals, even considering such a criterion for eliminating some patients from ICUs is unthinkable. They believe that everyone has the same right of access, regardless of the root of the problem. On the other hand, with a move towards more concern for the greater good, others believe that the bed should be given to someone with a greater likelihood of benefiting from it. This becomes even more of a social problem in a system that is supported financially by public money, as is the case universally in Canada and for those patients in the United States who qualify for government Medicare and Medicaid. Should the taxpayer have to bear the financial burden, which is quite substantial in ICUs, for those who fail to look after themselves? Evidently they should, because there is little move afoot in medical circles to treat these people any differently, at least in part because medical science does not allow physicians to determine accurately the extent to which particular risk factors contributed to the illness of any one individual.

The next question that needs to be examined is the length of time that a person should be treated in an ICU. Recent medical literature has referred to a new kind of patient: 'high-tech chronics,' are the creation of medical care itself, of the current love affair that medicine is having with technology. Although a demanding public and the media are partly to blame for this development, physicians need to accept responsibility for deceiving the public in allowing them to believe in the unfailing abilities of high-tech medicine (Hutchison 1988). The result is the problem of how to decide when to stop treating. 'The current approach ... is to remove patients from life-sustaining therapy only when it is in *their* best interest, never when it is solely in the best interest of another' (Truog 1992, 14). Although it is fairly well known that physicians do make decisions about rationing care before care is begun, it seems that, once a decision to treat is made, it is very difficult to stop on the basis of another patient's needs. Robert Truog, associate director of the neonatal intensive care unit at Children's Hospital in Boston, has also said, 'Rationing is a reality in the ICU. Studies indicate it is being performed without a clear idea of the principles and objectives that should underlie allocation decisions' (ibid., 16).

Dr Truog recognizes what some other physicians have failed to see – namely, that, while doctors are called upon to play an even greater part in the decisions that affect the rationing of health care resources, they have little background to prepare them for this task. The fact is that it is very difficult to predict how well an increasingly large number of patients will do with intensive care treatment. Therefore, it is sometimes a difficult task to decide which patients derive greater benefit medically from this level of care than others.

'TO DO NO HARM ...'

There is little doubt that ICU technology has been developed to benefit all of us. Many medical miracles would not occur today at all if not for the attention patients receive from nurses and doctors in modern ICUs. But, like everything else in medicine, those extreme measures don't come without potentially harmful side-effects.

A British professor of neurosurgery who is no stranger to the inner working of an intensive care unit has identified three ways that people are harmed by intensive care (Jennett 1984). First, he believes that patients who are not comatose and are aware of all that is going on around them may suffer as a result of the multitude of invasive procedures. Patients who are conscious while they are on ventilators, unable to speak because of the breathing tube, have said later how terrified they were.

The second harm caused by ICU is the loss of dignity that seems to go with the territory. The numerous procedures carried out by so many different types of health professionals contribute to this loss of dignity. So, too, does the actual physical set-up of many ICUs. Intensive care units in older hospitals and those that have not been renovated recently likely have the more traditional physical set-up whereby all patients are cared for in one very large room for ease of monitoring. With little privacy and only a thin curtain between the patient and the outside world, dignity is at a premium.

The final harm is a difficult one to document but involves the possibility of extending a life of poor quality, especially in situations where the patient's wishes are not even known. For many of us, a long life of poor quality is more harmful than a shorter life of high quality.

As health care consumers, we have to become more educated about both the scientific and the moral dimensions of care that is given in ICUs and the possible outcomes for the patients. Intensive care units are the tip of the health care resource-allocation iceberg. If society and the medical profession can deal with most visible issue, they might be able to devise a model on which to base the large body of unpleasant decisions that lurk beneath the surface of medical care.

As one writer put it, if we fail to look more critically at these issues and help the doctors to make some needed decisions, we run the risk of critical care units becoming the 'cemeteries of the future, populated by machine-maintained patients who are comatose and moribund, neither alive nor dead' (Cohen 1986, 41).

11

Making Babies ... The High-Tech Way

Dr Smart didn't usually treat infertility patients. Rather, she left
them to the obstetricians who specialized in those types of
things. This morning, however, she found herself responding to
a request that she consult on a case in the prenatal unit. The
obstetrician wanted Dr Smart to be familiar with this patient in
case complications arose and she ended up in the ICU.

Dr Smart read through the thick chart. Susan Forbes was
twenty-five years old and was six-months pregnant with her first
child. This young woman would now spend the remainder of
her pregnancy in the hospital because of a pre-existing medical
condition; she was a liver transplant recipient. At the age of
twenty-two, one year after her marriage and a month after she
had been told she would likely never have children, she suffered
massive liver failure and had been on the brink of death when a
donor liver became available and she received a transplant. Her
medical condition had been a bit unstable since that time, with
several episodes of rejection, all of which had been successfully
treated, but she continued on large doses of her anti-rejection
drugs.

Her young husband, a recent medical school graduate, had
been at her side through all of this, but had been devastated by
the earlier news that they could never have children. Susan
decided that they would not give up. At considerable expense,
she had approached an infertility clinic that had taken her on as
a patient. She had undergone *in vitro* fertilization and implanta-

tion, and now she was pregnant. Although a handful of liver transplant patients had successfully carried pregnancies and given birth to apparently healthy babies, most had been more stable than Susan. Complicating things further, a mild rejection crisis had begun to develop. Her own doctor was worried that her transplant might fail. Dr Smart closed the chart and spoke to one of the nurses who accompanied her to the patient's bedside.

It used to be fairly simple: Girl meets boy. Girl marries boy. Girl has baby. Girl reaches menopause and realizes that one of the advantages of 'the change' is the luxury of no longer having to consider the possibility of pregnancy. Times have changed.

The term 'reproductive technology' is in widespread use in both the academic medical press and the mass media. To put it simply, the term refers to the use of high-technology procedures in human reproduction. These technological procedures are designed to help a woman to conceive and carry a child through a pregnancy to birth.

A whole host of cultural and religious teachings surround pregnancy and childbirth. Add to these the rapid rate of scientific advancement in reproductive medicine, and we are left with a growing list of unanswered ethical questions that are becoming more high profile as each day passes.

THE PROBLEMS AND THE TECHNOLOGY

Before we can fully discuss the dilemmas that face physicians in the arena of reproductive technology, and the extent to which they have been able to deal with them, we need to discuss what reproductive problems exist today and the medical technology that has been applied to solve them.

Infertility
If there is any one issue that is inextricably entwined with reproductive technology of the 1990s, it is human infertility. Many a feminist author has alluded to the ludicrous aspects of birth control – that women spend years trying to ensure that

they do not have babies only to find out at some point in the future that they can't anyway.

The rate of infertility in developed countries has risen dramatically over the past quarter-century. While women age twenty to twenty-four have traditionally been considered to be in their most fertile years, the incidence of infertility among women in that age group rose 177 per cent between 1965 and 1982 (Wallis 1984). While there is no one single cause for this striking change, researchers have identified several factors, some of which are, themselves, the offspring of developments in modern medicine. Among these are the after-effects of some forms of contraception, including the birth control pill and intrauterine devices, as well as abortion. Other factors that contribute to infertility are the consequences and complications many women suffer following sexually transmitted diseases, such as chlamydia and gonorrhoea.

When couples discover that they are unable to conceive, they react with a variety of emotions. Some accept it as a fact of their lives; others are devastated. Infertility seems to put some people on an emotional roller coaster that includes feelings of shock, horror, anger, and denial. One infertility counsellor describes the impact of this discovery: 'Infertility rips at the couple's relationship; it affects sexuality, self-image, and self-esteem. It stalls careers, devastates life savings, and damages associations with friends and family' (Wallis 1984, 40). It is against this emotional backdrop that modern medicine presents couples with an array of technological approaches that are designed to give them hope. Along the way to fulfilling their dreams, the new technology becomes a double-edged sword, offering along with hope a host of confusing questions. While the advances give hope where none existed before, they can be very expensive and they do change the natural human processes.

Several notable approaches designed to deal with this inability to conceive have emerged. Their applications depend upon whether it is the mother or the father who is infertile, and what has caused the problem. For example, when the father's sperm count or quality is to blame, simple artificial insemination from donor sperm might be all that is necessary. As the situation becomes more complicated, numerous permutations and combinations of solutions are available, among them donor sperm and eggs, *in vitro* fertilization (the combination of egg and sperm outside the body under laboratory conditions), and sometimes the use of surrogate mothers. Clearly, these approaches represent procreation without benefit of sex, a concept that was once confined to the realm of science fiction.

While most doctors practising in this area work only in a highly ethical way, a few have provided reason for health care consumers to ask questions. In a now classic study reported in 1979, of the 400 doctors who practised artificial insemination using donor sperm, 80 per cent used sperm from medical students or residents almost exclusively. The researchers even found one practitioner who had used the same donor for some fifty pregnancies (Curie and Cohen 1979). There has long been a standing joke among medical students that a trip to the sperm bank would provide those few extra dollars for the weekend. While, on the surface, this might seem simply humorous, critics consider it to be a subtle form of eugenics – in other words, physicians exercising their power by controlling heredity.

This questionable activity was taken to fraudulent limits in 1992 when Dr Cecil B. Jacobson was charged in a fertility case that was widely reported in the media. A federal jury in Alexandria, Virginia, found him guilty of artificially inseminating more than a dozen patients with his own sperm, without the patients' knowledge that he was the donor. Imagine the patients' surprise when they looked closely at their new babies, only to find that the person the child resembled most was their fertility specialist! That is exactly what happened.

The New York Times report quoted Jacobson as saying, 'I spent my life trying to help women have children. If I felt I was a criminal or broke the law, I would never have done it' ('Doctor is found guilty ...' 1992, A 14:1). The fifty-five-year-old doctor, who is credited with introducing amniocentesis to the United States, was found by DNA testing to be the father of fifteen babies, and was linked to about seventy-five more. Despite the moral questions surrounding this use (or abuse) of power, there are no laws or clear-cut guidelines prohibiting doctors from taking such action. Dr Jacobson's mistake was that he led the patients to believe that the sperm was from anonymous donors, thus lying to them – a serious breach of trust in the doctor–patient relationship. Fortunately, it is a rare occurrence.

The whole area of *in vitro* fertilization has been the centre of considerable ethical debate within the medical profession, as well among the public, and the issues are still unresolved. Recent studies indicate that only about 15 per cent of infertile couples are successfully treated with this method. One writer says this about the process: 'In vitro fertilization is costly, labor intensive, inconvenient, and has only limited success. Is it fair to society to offer a treatment with such a low return rate?' (Bain n. d.). For those people successfully treated, however, the children born to them seem to add immeasurably to their lives.

Sex Preselection

In spite of attempts to identify male and female sperm and to have the selected ones unite with an egg to produce an offspring of the desired sex, the only way to effectively preselect the sex of your baby at present is by selective abortion. The success of selecting the sex of your offspring is directly related to the ability of medical science, first, to determine the sex of a fetus long before birth, and, second, to abort a fetus of undesired sex. Apart from the controversy that still swirls around the abortion issue, the idea of being able to select the sex of your babies has its own problems.

Currently, there are basically three ways that medical science can determine the sex of a fetus. Keep in mind that the primary medical use of these procedures is to identify medical problems in the fetus, not to determine sex. The first, and least invasive, is ultrasound. After sixteen weeks of gestation, the sex of the fetus can be determined by routine ultrasound. A transvaginal ultrasound can determine the sex of a baby at approximately twelve to fourteen weeks, although it is not a foolproof method. Determination of the baby's sex by ultrasound is often simply a by-product of the fact that the mother is having an ultrasound anyway. If it is crucial to know the sex of the child, other methods that examine the genetic material of the fetus must be used. These include amniocentesis and chorionic villus sampling (CVS).

Amniocentesis is carried out after the thirteenth week of pregnancy. This, in itself poses serious problems, as it is too late for the simplest approaches to abortion. CVS, on the other hand, can be done safely at ten to twelve weeks, but it is still done primarily only in large teaching hospitals and carries with it a risk of abnormalities in the development of the fetus' limbs if done earlier than ten weeks. In *in vitro* fertilization, the sex of the pre-embryo can be determined, and only the chosen sex implanted in the mother and allowed to develop to term.

At first glance, it might seem to you to be an advantage to be able to select the sex of your babies. You might be happier if you had the boy or the girl you had longed for, as the argument goes, and would be a better parent. You could even out your family, instead of having two children of the same sex. Or, you could try to avoid sex-linked hereditary disease, such as haemophilia, usually found in males, by selecting female babies. However, the arguments against the practice are equally compelling.

Most of these counter-arguments are based on the widespread (and well-documented) belief that there is a preference for boys, particularly for the first-born and if the family is going to have only one child. Some of the arguments that have been advanced are:

- In general, allowing people free rein to select the sex of their offspring would result in an unbalancing of the sex ratio.
- Assuming that there would likely be a preference for males, the result would be a diminishing of the status of women.
- Based on the belief that parents would generally prefer their first born to be male (Wertz and Fletcher 1989), an unbalancing of the birth order would result, with serious psychological and legal ramifications. Many psychologists and others believe that birth order affects people's psychological make-

up. In addition, it can be very important in legal issues, especially those related to inheritance.

As is the case in many ethical problems, in one particular situation only one answer might be the right one, while in terms of
the effects on society as a whole, a different answer might be
appropriate. Knowing the facts and thinking beyond the rights of
the individual enable consumers to help governments and doctors decide where to draw the line.

Embryo Research

A third issue is the emerging area of research on the human
embryo. When eggs and sperm are united in a petri dish in a laboratory to form human embryos, often more embryos are created than are required for the particular clinical application,
such as implantation in an infertile woman's uterus or in a surrogate. Thus, there is the ever larger question of what to do with
these extra embryos. Do we destroy them? Do we freeze them?
Do we use them for research? The last option is a temptation for
many researchers and, although many health-related organizations worldwide have developed guidelines for people involved
in this kind of research, it is unclear whether all researchers
abide by them.

There are some specific concerns in this area. The first relates
to the issue of consent. As we have discussed previously, you as a
patient have the right to decide what will be done to your body
by medical science. When it comes to human embryos outside
the body, however, it is very unclear whether the person who
gave the ova (the woman), the person who provided the sperm
(the man), the person who joined the two together (the doctor),
or someone else (for example, the state) has the right of owner-
ship. As for the question of who has any rights at all regarding
the disposal of the embryos, neither the law nor medical ethics
has the answer at this time.

The second area of ethical concern has more to do with the
nature of the actual research itself. The question is: when do you
stop nurturing the embryo as it develops into a human fetus?

When does the fetus become a person? The American Fertility Society believes that it is permissible to experiment on the human embryo up until the fourteenth day of development (Hill 1986). At that time, the nervous system really begins to develop, and the embryo normally implants in the uterus. Although the permissibility is not legally determined, it is an educated scientific judgment.

Fetal Therapy

Evolving from any discussion of how human embryos should be treated in medical science is a set of problems associated with fetal therapy. It is now possible to treat a variety of disorders that can be detected *in utero*, long before the baby is actually born. This is a very interesting development in the face of generalized tolerance for abortion. It is this conflict of the rights – those of the woman versus those of the unborn child – that leads to many of the ethical questions surrounding fetal therapy.

At the same time as medical science has developed better and safer ways for women to have abortions and they have become more widely available, new and better ways to treat the fetus before birth have emerged. On the one hand, some doctors are treating the fetus as no more than an extension of the woman's body. Others treat the fetus as if it were a human being with the right to safe medical treatment. As a result, physicians who disagree among themselves have been unable to help women or society to come to terms with these conflicting values. For example, in Canada, the Medical Research Council guidelines tell us that it is unacceptable to harm or mutilate a fetus. On the other hand, it is acceptable to abort one. The scientific validity of some of the procedures suggested by researchers cannot help but be questioned.

WHAT YOU CAN DO

Even if you never face directly the issues surrounding the use of reproductive technology, as a concerned and educated health care consumer you can help to answer some of the questions that will be put to North Americans over the next decade. As we have looked at the marvels that medical science has to offer in these areas, we have alluded to some of the attendant problems. You can help to solve them.

Reproductive technology is an issue that affects women more than it does men. It affects their bodies, their emotions, their thinking. While many of the members of the medical profession argue that these applications of medical science lead to more freedom to make decisions about reproductive issues for women, many feminists argue that they instead lead to *reproductive enslavement*. In part, this opinion stems from the notion that, if we all had control of the sex of our offspring, the percentage of women in the population would likely drop. The eventual outcome would be that women would be prized by society for their reproductive capacity and would be less likely to be prized for anything else.

It seems that, for many modern parents, children are valued, not for themselves, but for what they can add to their parents' lives. This *commodification of children* makes them little different from a new car or taking a vacation. When children become commodities, people seek to acquire them in the same way they would other 'valuable' possessions.

As North American society looks at children as commodities, there is a need, not only to have them in the first place, but to make sure that they are as 'perfect' as possible. As technology advances, we come ever closer to being able to 'engineer' the perfect child. Parents who choose one child over another, for whatever reason, are making a decision that contributes to an intolerance for those deemed 'less perfect' according to some arbitrary standard. Those who are unable to tolerate a particular characteristic in an offspring will be unlikely to be able to tolerate it in a stranger.

Another general problem associated with reproductive technologies is that there is *unequal access*. Such technologies are often not considered to be part of a basic level of care, and some procedures, such as sex preselection, are offered only at expensive clinics to which only the well-off can come for help. Joan Rothschild, a professor of political science at the University of

Lowell in Massachusetts, says that the people who typically make use of these medical approaches in the United States are white, upper middle class, with less tolerance for handicapped children than those of lesser means and of minority extraction (1991). What this means for the future is that most children with disabilities, now and in adulthood, are likely to be clustered in the lower socio-economic levels of society. Who is going to care for these people who cannot care for themselves? Sex preselection may be one of the most striking examples in medical science of what might happen if there is a failure to look at the long-term good of society as opposed to the current good for one individual patient or family.

Finally, we come to the general concern about the rights of the woman versus the rights of the unborn child. We have already discussed modern society's love affair with 'rights' movements. Alongside all of the other rights movements is an emerging interest in the rights of the unborn. This is a result of medical science's innovations.

While there is no universally accepted cut-off point, doctors often refer to the twentieth to twenty-fifth week of pregnancy as the time when the fetus could actually live outside the womb. Survival rates for these babies, however, vary considerably. From a legal point of view, where the fetus used to be looked upon entirely as an integral part of the mother, recent opinions are reflecting a shift towards thinking that sees the fetus as having rights too. This has a number of consequences for pregnant women.

If a woman knowingly harms her unborn child through neglect of her health – for example, by continuing to abuse drugs – does that make her legally liable for damage to the child? Does a doctor have a moral responsibility to do something to protect that unborn child? You have to look at the situation from both the mother's and the unborn child's perspective to determine what you believe to be right.

Society will have to come to a general consensus on these issues to help doctors who will continue to use the technology to push the limits of life to the extreme until they are told by society to stop.

12

Every Baby Has Its Chance: Neonatal Intensive Care

Alan and Barbara K. had been looking forward to the birth of their first child for a long time. They had put off parenthood until they were ten years into marriage and had firmly established their financial and emotional framework. Finally, in June, Barbara bought a pregnancy-test kit at the drugstore on her way home from work one Friday afternoon, and on Saturday morning she crept out of bed before Alan had even awakened.

She followed the directions carefully and, by the time the test was completed, she had confirmed what she had suspected for some weeks. She and Alan were going to be parents in about eight months. When she woke Alan, they shared the same feelings of both happiness and terror but decided, in the end, that happiness won out. So they went about their business for the next two months, deciding to leave baby preparations until the eighth month of the pregnancy. Giving birth was the last thing on Barbara's mind one fall afternoon when she began experiencing pain while she was reading a story to her first-graders. Later, the blood stains were an ominous sign.

She called Alan, terrified about what might happen. He tore home and they raced to the hospital. Despite all efforts to stop it, Barbara gave birth twenty hours later to a tiny baby girl who weighed in at just under two pounds. At that moment, both Barbara and Alan knew that the certainty they had felt about becoming parents was tenuous indeed. This case presents every pregnant couple's worst nightmare, and the odds in favour of this baby's survival were poor. They were, however, much better than they would have been had she been born twenty-five years ago.

In spite of the odds against these tiny babies and others with life-threatening problems at the time of their births, the philosophy of the doctors and nurses who care for these tiny creatures can be summed up by one nurse's belief about her work: 'Every baby has its chance.' And so it goes.

Although this philosophy may seem simple and straightforward, it is not as simple as diagnosing a sick baby, treating that child, and evaluating the outcome. Questions of when to treat, how to treat, and when to stop treating are coupled with perplexing concerns in modern medicine about such things as who should be making these decisions and whether or not we can afford this aggressive approach to grave illness with uncertain outcomes. Despite the fact that neonatal intensive care as a specialty is not much more than twenty years old, it has spawned an enormous number of as yet unanswered questions.

TO TREAT OR NOT TO TREAT?

The brief history of neonatal intensive care is a good example of medical technology that has advanced at a far greater speed than our ability to deal with the moral dilemmas it presents both to the medical profession and to society. At the beginning of this century, when every birth was a home birth, a baby born too early or too ill to survive on its own simply died. After the Second World War, significant advances in the care of severely ill babies were just beginning to be made, and developments such as new plastics and antibiotics contributed greatly to these endeavours. These advances, the forerunners of some of the basic care that is given in neonatal intensive care units today, included feeding babies through tubes into their stomachs, and incubators that provide a sort of plastic bubble environment for the neonate. In 1975 neonatology became a board-certified specialty in the United States.

Doctors who treat severely ill babies are faced with three fundamental questions:

- When do we treat these babies?
- When do we not treat these babies?
- When do we stop treating these babies?

And these are not the only questions. Others include how aggressively the chosen treatment should be applied and which treatment should be used.

None of these questions has a straightforward answer because no one can predict with accuracy in many cases whether or not the treatment will do any good. The results might be a live child who suffers from a variety of problems, including cerebral palsy, mental retardation, blindness, and learning disabilities. Until the 1960s, severely ill babies were simply allowed to die, and neither the news media nor the general public really gave the matter much consideration.

The first two questions are best considered together: when do we treat and when do we not treat? If it is your own baby, the answer is quite different from the one arrived at with some measure of objectivity. Although it might be easy to simply say that, based on the North American ethic of protecting the sanctity of life, every baby should be treated, doctors are more realistic than that. Using that basis for the decision would mean that, in every medical circumstance, regardless of the known futility of the therapy or its likely adverse effects, severely ill babies should be treated. In real terms, the question becomes: how do we know when therapy will be futile, and would treatment be more harmful than helpful in the long term? An additional concern is whether resources being channelled into the treatment of one very sick newborn would not be better used to ensure better prenatal care, hot lunches, or a variety of other things to improve the life and health of many more children.

In 1983, a coalition of American organizations that are concerned with the ethical treatment of very sick new babies issued a statement of principles to help doctors, parents, and governments come to grips with the difficulty of making decisions about when to treat and when not to treat. These guidelines included the following:

- If the medical care would be beneficial, it should be provided. Even if the child is likely to have future disabilities, these should play no part in making the decision to treat or not to treat.
- Once a decision has been made to treat, society, including medicine and the governments, have a responsibility to make the resources available for as long as is necessary (O'Neill 1983).

The first guideline is clear in its conviction that neither doctors nor parents are in a position to make judgments about the future quality of life for these children. This is particularly problematic for society in light of the implications of the second guideline, which is related to the issue of resource availability. As one medical writer has said, 'One predictable consequence of more aggressive treatment, and the resulting increase in the number of survivors with varying degrees of handicap, is increasing costs for society' (Zupancic 1992, 1073). It seems, then, that the medical profession is looking in one direction for answers to these dilemmas, and citizens' groups are looking in another.

In the United States, federal law requires doctors to treat all sick babies unless it is clear from a medical point of view that they would not benefit. This legislation considers the issue of medical futility, and comes in the form of the 1985 amendments to the Child Abuse and Neglect Prevention and Treatment Act. As a consequence of laws like this, many neonatologists report that they treat infants whom they really feel should not be treated (Rostain and Bhutani 1989). There is no legal guidance, however, to direct the decision of when to stop treatment. That decision becomes a medical judgment coupled with an ethical one.

The decision to treat or not to treat sick babies in sophisticated medical facilities is not based on universally accepted ethical principles. Unfortunately, neither is it based on known quantities about the outcomes of medical procedures. The decisions are made on a case-by-case basis. The issue of quality of life does, however, play a part when the decision making is left up to members of the medical profession.

When the medical profession examines what is meant by the term 'quality of life,' they use guidelines such as the activity level of the individual, whether or not a person can or has the potential to care for him or herself, general health, social support systems, and the individual's outlook on life. While these are not directly applicable to the situation with sick babies, there have been suggestions that, if these were projected into the future, some measure of quality of life might be available. Unfortunately, one person's quality of life is another person's living hell. It is very subjective, no matter what scale you use.

The question of when you decide to stop treatment is particularly worrisome. With a medical profession socialized the way it has been for most of this century, once a decision is made to treat a patient the decision to stop is even more difficult. It is almost as if they say, 'We have come this far; let us go on.' Sometimes the result is not the prolongation of life, but the prolongation of dying.

The use of labels is another issue of concern. Health care workers are notorious for their use of labels, and these very sick babies are prime targets for some of the most widespread ones. These babies are often referred to as 'hopelessly ill,' 'non-viable,' 'terminal.' As one writer put it, 'the meaning of these phrases is often vague and they can have powerful effects on decisions, becoming self-fulfilling prophecies' (Fost 1981, 234). It can be frightening to the uninitiated layperson to hear such terms bandied about in general conversation by doctors and nurses. It does not necessarily indicate lack of respect for their patients, only a helplessness at having no other words to use to describe the futility of the medical treatment. Futility in patient care is powerlessness for the doctor.

WHO SHOULD MAKE THESE DECISIONS?

The question of who should make these decisions is an especially important one, since the one person who is most directly affected by the decision – the baby – does not have the capacity to make it. At present, there are several other possibilities for who *does* and who *should* make those decisions, but these are not necessarily the same people in all circumstances.

There are several parties who do assist in making such decisions and who could potentially help:

- Clearly, the child's parents are important. During such an emotional time, however, they often defer to the medical staff, whose interests go beyond this one patient to other things like the reputation of the institution and teaching opportunities.
- The medical and nursing staff involved should provide the parents with adequate information to make decisions. This responsibility does not, however, extend to forcing their own personal values on the parents. It might require them to help the parents to see the bigger picture, including the future of their child, and the resources that are required both now and in an uncertain future. All health care decisions have lasting consequences.
- Whether we like it or not, governments currently do and will continue to play a part, indirect though it may be, in the decision to treat very sick babies. Often their input will relate to the issue of economics. It is extremely expensive to treat sick newborns and, as time goes on, health care system gatekeepers will face ever more frequently the question of where the money will be taken from.

Parents need help from both doctors and others who are experienced in dealing with ethical problems in health care. If we agree that the parents have the most crucial role to play in these decisions about their children, then the question remains: can the parents make a truly informed, free decision at a time of such emotional upheaval? Is it even fair to ask them to do so?

Medicine is not an exact science, but a combination of applied science and the human act of caring. Care of very sick infants is one of the many areas of medicine where cutting-edge science meets the human component. Thus, the decision making in this area needs to reflect the collaborative model that we discussed at the beginning of this book. Both the doctors and the parents need to assess the situation and come together with their own perspectives. Only in this atmosphere of understanding and cooperation will we be able to make decisions in the best interests of everyone involved.

13

New Organs for Old:
Organ Replacement Technology

Dr Smart was having a busy day. For many others it might have seemed unduly stressful, but Dr Smart thrived on the constant demands on her time and expertise, and the sometimes unforeseen situations that popped up between planned events. She was now rushing to the surgical intensive care unit to answer a page from the head nurse.

Mr Johnston, the forty-seven-year-old patient she was on her way to see, had been admitted to the ICU following a liver transplant to which he had reluctantly submitted. It was now two weeks later, and the liver transplant surgeon had put Mr Johnston's name back on the list for another new liver since the first transplant was failing. When the head nurse found out that this man had been placed back on the transplant list, she was concerned – in fact, he was flabbergasted, and she told Dr Smart so just minutes earlier on the telephone. The head nurse indicated that, as of this morning, Mr Johnston's body was rejecting his new liver and he was suffering from the consequences of massive doses of the drugs that sometime stop this rejection process. These consequences involved the breakdown of the body's ability to fight off infections, and he was growing a variety of micro-organisms in his bloodstream, lungs, and bone marrow. He was dying.

The head nurse's experience told her that he would never survive another onslaught of drugs to suppress further his immune system. In addition, his current infection made him an especially bad candidate for surgery. Given this outlook, the transplantation of another liver into this man would result in the loss of a chance for another person. The transplant surgeon was not, however, to be deterred. The head nurse had decided to confer with Dr Smart in her capacity as head of the intensive care units.

Dr Smart arrived in the unit and was updated by both the head nurse and the surgical resident. When the surgeon arrived, she discussed the case with him, and it was his opinion that, since the man's liver was being rejected, he was a candidate for another transplant. While they were conferring, the transplant coordinator rushed up to inform the surgeon that a donor was available. There was no patient other than Mr Johnston of the same blood type in need of a liver in this hospital, but a transplant program in a neighbouring state had said that they would take it. The transplant surgeon decided to keep it, and Mr Johnston was transplanted. Six days later he died of a lung complication that had been present before the transplant, but his liver was functioning. As the old saying goes, the operation was a success but the patient died.

Over the past twenty years, they have made the headlines more often than any other single group of medical professionals, despite the fact that an infinitesimally small percentage of our population ever receives their services. Their media story is a journalist's dream. It has human drama, heroism, pathos, grief, human suffering, high technology, medical breakthroughs, and, perhaps even more compelling from a journalist's perspective, controversy – both moral and, from time to time, legal. They are all this and more. They are the transplant doctors. But this view of them is changing.

Somewhere along the way, on their road to creating these 'patchwork people,' as their patients have been called, the evangelical approach to their work has caused some people, both within and outside the field, to turn sour. Two individuals who spent many years working with health professionals in the field of organ transplantation recognize in these professionals the following characteristics: 'a rescue-oriented, often zealous determination to maintain life at any cost; and a relentless, hubris-ridden refusal to accept limits' (Fox and Swazey 1992, 10). This is the side of organ transplantation that the public rarely sees.

Since it is the heroic, medical miracle aspect of transplantation, coupled with heart-wrenching pleas for organ donation, that so often makes the headlines, we are going to take you on a quite different trip through the halls of the transplant units. While we do not dispute the enormous good that has come of the research and practice in this field, the fact remains that the increasingly complex ethical dilemmas that are part and parcel of human organ and tissue transplantation have been considered from time to time by the practitioners but haven't even come close to being solved. Since only a small number of us will truly require replacement of our organs but all of us are being asked to recycle the ones we have and sign donor cards, it is only fitting that we give equal time to the unresolved dilemmas in the field.

In a distinctly different case that was given high-profile coverage in the media, a mother and father came head to head with the attitudes of modern medical science when they refused to let the surgeons replace their baby son's failing liver with a transplant. At the age of three months, baby K'aila was diagnosed with terminal liver failure, his only hope for physical survival a liver transplant. K'aila's parents refused this treatment, which has a success rate of 80 to 85 per cent but requires long-term follow-up and treatment with drugs to suppress the immune system. Since their decision was not well received by the doctor, they found another who respected their wishes.

Their refusal of the transplant made headlines and impelled the paediatrician to report them to the Department of Social Services, which made an application to the courts for custody of the baby so that the transplant could be carried out (pending a suitable organ being available, of course). The long and painful process in the courts finally resulted in a decision that upheld the parents' right to make such a decision on behalf of their child.

K'aila's mother, a Native American, told her story in an issue of the ethics journal *Humane Medicine.* 'As Native American people, whose cultural and spiritual traditions are steeped in a reverence for the wisdom inherent in the Creator's natural order, we felt we might be committing a grave error if we tried to recreate our son's body. It seemed obvious that, while trying to play at being God, we would run the risk of violating K'aila's spiritual as well as physical identity' (Paulette 1993, 14).

THE HISTORY OF A PHENOMENON

While many of the uninitiated may believe that organ transplantation is the product of twentieth-century medical scientific thinking, the idea itself is not new at all. The idea of using one person's tissue – namely, blood – for another can be traced back as far as the fifteenth century; historians believe that blood was actually transfused into Pope Innocent in 1490. Although initially planned to be a live-donor tissue transplant, as we would have called it today, it actually turned out to be a cadaveric tissue transplant. The donors, the three young boys from whom the blood was taken, subsequently died, but then so did the pope, resulting in the swift departure of the surgeon from the country. Also during the fifteenth century, historical references to attempts to transplant teeth from cadavers have been found.

While the idea of transplanting organs has surfaced again and again throughout the history of medicine since that time, the era of what is now modern transplant medicine was ushered in near the beginning of the twentieth century. In fact, one of the earliest recorded kidney transplants was carried out in 1902, and the problems experienced by the patient were to be repeated again and again until medical science began to learn something about the body's immune system. What they didn't know at the turn of the century was that, if you transplant a foreign body, in this case a kidney, into a human being, the recipient will develop antibodies, the body's attempt to ward off what it recognizes as foreign and potentially harmful. Until medical scientists had a handle on not only this system within the body but also methods to reduce this natural response, which we know as 'the rejection response,' transplantation was doomed to failure.

The first successful kidney transplant was carried out in Boston in 1954. Although the science of immunology was still not very advanced, the success was a result of the fact that the donor was the identical twin brother of the recipient. With a DNA pattern shared with his brother, the recipient's body did not recognize the kidney as being foreign, and thus did not reject it. This is what we refer to as a 'living-related donor transplant,' a form of transplantation which continues today. It is used primarily because of a scarcity of cadaveric donors. Since we can live well with only one healthy kidney and we are born with two, the notion of a live donor is very appealing.

Over the next several decades, major strides were made in the surgical techniques of transplantation. The real success story of modern transplantation, however, is the development of methods to suppress the normal immune response of the human body. This allows non-identical tissue to be accepted. Today, kidneys are still the most frequently transplanted solid organ, but many other types of transplantation are almost as commonplace. These include the liver, heart, and lung, along with some transplantation of the pancreas and parts of the gastrointestinal system, stomach, and bowel. In addition, combinations of these organs are also transplanted with varying degrees of success, the most notable being the heart–lung transplant.

On 2 December 1992, transplant programs celebrated a quarter of a century since Dr Christiaan Barnard performed the first human-heart transplant in South Africa. He grafted the heart of a twenty-four-year-old woman who was fatally injured in a traffic accident into the chest of fifty-four-year-old Louis Washansky, who was dying of end-stage heart failure. Although the patient died of pneumonia eighteen days later, this marked the beginning of fast and furious development in the field. Apart from being the first human-heart transplant, the case was a watershed of a different kind.

Until that time, kidneys had been hurriedly removed from donors moments after the cessation of heartbeat, the moment when death was thought to have occurred. The success of a heart transplant, however, relied on the availability of a heart that was beating and thus had a blood supply until only shortly before it was removed from the body. Before this time, it was widely accepted that this act of organ retrieval would cause death. This put into clinical practice the new research findings and beliefs about human death – namely, that the death of the brain is the only real way to determine death.

Despite the fact that the patient died, the great contribution that Dr Barnard made to the field was that he moved heart transplantation from the laboratory to the clinical setting and set in motion incredible interest in solving the myriad clinical problems besetting the field. The primary problem that he brought to the surface was how to declare patients dead when their hearts were still beating.

Throughout the 1970s and into the 1980s, the search for ways to solve the rejection problems continued. While there were drugs available to reduce this bodily response, most had unpleasant side-effects, to the point of toxicity. The most serious research in the field focused on finding drugs that would stop the rejection without causing even greater problems for the patients.

By the early 1980s, the success rate for kidney transplantation was about 50 to 55 per cent for one year, with 3 to 5 per cent of those grafts failing each year thereafter. At that time, a new drug was introduced. Although not without its own side-effects, this drug, cyclosporin A, had a remarkable effect on the transplant patients who received it, and within three years of its routine use, success rates for kidney transplantation were reported to be in the vicinity of 80 to 85 per cent for one year. This was a remarkable medical-scientific achievement.

As cyclosporin began to be used for patients receiving a wide variety of organs, their success rates also climbed. In recent years, even more impressive drug therapy has arrived on the scene, and the outlook is even more positive.

That is the good news in the development of organ transplantation. However, this is one of those stories in which the success of the endeavour has been materially responsible for its problems. The primary problem that has plagued transplantation from the outset, has never improved, and is getting worse every time we recognize that more people could benefit from transplantation, is the shortage of donors. There never have been, are not at present, and are likely never to be enough organs to go around. Therein lies the crux of most of the ethical problems that continue to swirl around this field.

ETHICS AND ORGAN DONORS

Hippocrates could never have imagined the multitude of difficult ethical problems that have developed as a consequence of success in the field of organ replacement. What would the Father of Medicine have said about the idea that others may actually have a 'right' to our organs when we no longer need them? What would he have said about paying people for their organs? The list of questions goes on and on.

Only about 2 per cent of people who die each year in North America die in a way that makes them suitable organ donors. These criteria include:

- They must die in a hospital of a significant injury to the brain.
- The criteria for determining 'brain death' must be applied and found to be met.
- After declaration of brain death, the patient must have a stable pulse and blood pressure maintained until the organs are removed.
- The patient must be free of infection, including hepatitis and HIV.
- Usually the patient must have no history of cancer.
- The patient must have been generally healthy until death.

Some centres also have age-related criteria. For example, older people are usually not suitable heart donors, but in some instances they may be used as kidney donors. In any case, it is clear that the population of potential donors is limited and, given the fact that many people do not sign organ donor cards and many families refuse to sign consent for donation or are never asked at all when the opportunity presents itself, the number of organ donors is dismal, to say the least. This is the reason that so many people must wait for donor organs. For example, the American Heart Association estimates that between 10 and 40 per cent of people awaiting heart transplantation die before a suitable heart is found ('Possible hearts for donation ...' 1992). It is this fact of not enough resources to treat everyone that has resulted in searches for other sources of donors and in the necessity for difficult decisions to be made about allocation.

As we turn to the specific areas where examination of the medical profession's ethical approaches is warranted, the first stop is an area that we have discussed in other contexts – that is, the problems associated with consent. The problem of informed decision making in the area of organ donation is multifaceted. Let us begin by examining the situation in which families of organ donors are approached for consent to donation.

Carol Kowalsky is a seventeen-year-old girl who was admitted to the intensive care unit with a severe head injury following a car accident on the night of her senior prom. Despite the surgical efforts to remove clots and ease pressure, she has succumbed to her injury and has been declared brain dead. These tests for brain death are being performed as her parents arrive, terrified for their daughter's life. They can hardly believe that the beautiful young woman of whom they snapped pictures just hours earlier was now lying motionless and battered beneath the sheets while a machine at her side breathes for her. Her parents' first reaction is denial – this can't be happening; it is their worst nightmare. They refuse to believe that she may be gone for good. The neurosurgeon who operated on Carol has just told them that she is clinically brain dead and that she would be a suitable organ donor, should they wish to consent. The only problem now is that her blood pressure is unstable and they will have to make a decision quickly. They are overwrought and refuse.

This scenario is not all that uncommon. People confronted by the death of a loved one refuse organ donation for a variety of reasons, ranging from fear of bodily mutilation to fear that a signed organ donor card might mean the medical staff will be less likely to do everything possible to save the donor's life in favour of someone else's. Although neither of these fears has any foundation in reality, each is a problem organ donor teams face every day. The ethical problem here is the question of whether, under these circumstances of emotional stress, a family can make a well-informed decision. Clearly, family discussion and decisions beforehand would help, but the fact remains that most people do not consider these matters before they become a reality. It is difficult for these situations not to be viewed by critics as coercive, especially if any members of the actual transplant team are involved in obtaining consent, as is the procedure in some places.

The other problem with consent for organ donation is the fact that many health professionals find it a very difficult question to ask at all, and therefore would rather avoid it entirely. Not asking the question could be considered as unethical as asking it under inappropriate circumstances. By avoiding the question, the health professional has placed his or her discomfort above the family's right to be offered the opportunity to make such a gift to another. In a number of jurisdictions in both Canada and the United States, the matter has been taken out of the hands of the medical personnel by the enactment of laws stipulating that all families in these circumstances should be asked, unless a specific situation makes it unsuitable to do so. Consequences of failure of the doctor to ask the question is a reduction in government insurance payments to the hospital involved.

The next ethical problem area in transplantation is the question of the morality of paying people for their organs. Commercial trade in organs in North America is illegal. Having said that, there are still questions about its morality. When cadaveric donors are in short supply and there are people willing to sell their organs, why do some medical personnel seem to have trouble with the concept? There are several objections. The primary one seems to be that the notion of payment would change the relationship between doctor and patient, and that there is a distinct possibility of using those who need the money most as donors for those who have the most resources and are able to pay. But there are other, more fundamental questions.

What is the human body worth? For many years, medical students were told that the body, a repository of a number of cheap chemicals, was worth very little – about $0.95, in fact. A recent article in *Family Practice*, a newspaper for family physicians, discussed a new book titled *Selling Yourself to Science*, by Jim Hogshire. According to Hogshire, our bodies are a veritable wealth of resources, many of which could have hefty price tags: a pint of blood has a resale value in the United States of $120; a cup of bone marrow is worth $10,000; a kidney should be worth $20,000 to $50,000; and the list goes on. In fact, he believes that our bodies should be considered to be a part of our estates and should be sold to provide money for our grieving relatives (Sutherland 1993). Hogshire's view is not shared by many in the medical profession who are willing to make their views known publicly. The International Transplantation Society is opposed to commercial trade in organs, but interest in it continues as the pool of available organs dwindles.

The next set of ethical concerns relates to the use of living persons as donors for organs. Obviously, we are talking about those organs that we can live without, like a second kidney or, more recently, a part of a liver. Until just a few years ago, the vast majority of live-donor transplants were kidneys from living relatives with a close tissue match to the recipient. Then, the shortage of cadaveric donors, coupled with advancements in the ability to suppress the immune response, made the idea of using unrelated living donors much more attractive. In Canada, this began with what has been termed 'emotionally related donors,' usually a husband and wife.

There are two types of ethical problems faced here. First, do transplant surgeons have the right to refuse to use consenting adults as donors, regardless of their relationship to the recipient? Second, do these surgeons have a right to subject healthy people to the risks posed by the surgery to remove the organ in question? The questions of doing good and doing no harm clearly come into conflict in these situations, and doctors continue to solve them on an *ad hoc* basis with no generally agreed-upon guidelines. As you travel from transplant centre to transplant centre, you will find that the rules, values, and practices vary considerably.

Another area of increasing media attention in the field of transplantation deals, not with the grafting of solid organs, but with the use of tissue – in this case, the use of tissue obtained from aborted fetuses. The main concern about fetal tissue is not its projected uses, which include the treatment of Parkinson's disease at the present time, and Alzheimer's disease and diabetes in the future, but about the source of the tissue. Aligned as they are with the abortion debate, the ethical concerns about fetal tissue transplantation revolve around the lack of general consensus about the following:

- Who has the right to give consent?
- Is it appropriate to view a pregnancy as utilitarian, allowing a woman to become pregnant for the sole purpose of providing a loved one with tissue?
- On the other hand, is it ethical to dispose of aborted tissue when it could be used for beneficial purposes?

Scientific research and subsequent advances in treatment approaches continue in organ transplantation while the ethical questions multiply. In fact, according to a widely reported study carried out at the University of Toronto Centre for Bioethics, one-third of the family physicians surveyed agreed that it would be acceptable to time an abortion to ensure optimum tissue for transplantation, 5 per cent had no objection to planning a pregnancy solely for the purposes of obtaining tissue, and 10 per cent thought it acceptable to mention the possibility of fetal tissue donation to women who were undecided about the abortion and then to give those who agreed priority in scheduling the procedure ('Abortions should be manipulated ...' 1992; Weber 1992).

Another high-profile area of concern is the movement towards the use of animals as organ donors for humans. Although this has largely been the domain of the research scientist, as advances are made in the suppression of the immune response it becomes more and more likely that this approach may have some clinical merit in the future. Until now, the attempts to transplant animal, principally baboon, organs into human beings have been experimental only.

The media drew the first public attention to this effort in 1984 when American surgeon Dr Leonard Bailey, of Loma Linda Medical Center in California, carried out what was believed to be the first implantation of a baboon heart into a terminally ill infant. The 'Baby Fae' case, as it came to be known in the media, was widely thought of as a clinical experiment on a defenceless infant, albeit a terminally ill one. Aside from the issue of transplanting the animal organ into a human being and all that entails both physiologically and morally, one fact of this particular situation that was not widely known was that, according to media reports, the baby inadvertently received a heart from a baboon whose blood group was incompatible. Dr Bailey publicly admitted the mistake after the fiasco. Interest in these 'xenografts,' as they are properly termed, waned for a time after this incident, but, in 1987, the issue was discussed in some depth at the International Transplantation Conference in Pittsburgh, ushering in an era of renewed interest. In June 1992, surgeons at the University of Pittsburgh Medical Center transplanted a baboon liver into a thirty-five-year-old man whose liver had failed because of hepatitis B, which is believed to have no effect on a baboon liver. This young man died in September, less than three months after the surgery, of what was found on autopsy to be an intracranial hemorrhage, and they confirmed that the man was HIV positive. The head of the transplant program pointed out at the time that the liver was in good shape. Perhaps once again the operation was a success, but the patient died.

In early 1993, the director of the largest transplant program in Canada, located in London, Ontario, announced that he was the principal investigator in a major study that would investigate the use of animals as organ donors. The $150,000 grant for the study was provided by Sandoz Canada, Inc., a pharmaceutical company (the one that manufactures cyclosporin, the anti-rejection drug). The first stage of the study will involve the transplantation of livers and kidneys between baboons and monkeys, but transplantation of animal organs into humans could begin as early as six months to a year later (Johnston 1993).

One final area that needs to be examined in light of its ethical components is the role of the media in the organ-donation process. Without a doubt, there is a need for the mass media to play a part in disseminating the message about the need for organ donors. The public at large is the source of the raw materials necessary for this medical treatment approach to become a reality. Problems arise, however, from the nature of the media reports.

Reporters and editors in the mass media have criteria that they use to determine the newsworthiness of an event or a person. Among these are timeliness, proximity, prominence, consequence, rarity and human interest (Hough 1988). And one other characteristic is controversy. What this means is that a relative non-story can become a story if it is happening now, it is happening in the neighbourhood of the readers or viewers, it involves prominent people or events, it will have impact on the community, it doesn't happen to everyone, and it has enough human drama to hook an audience. Thus, the stories about organ donation that have appeared in mass media have encompassed the following:

- the politician's child who needs an organ (prominence);
- the child who needs an organ but who has been turned down by the transplant program because of reasons judged by the reporter to be socially related (controversy and human drama);
- the child or adult who suffers from a very unusual illness (rarity);
- the pleas of the family members who have a loved one who needs an organ and who know enough about the process of mass media or enough people to get attention.

The first three relate to the media outlet's judgment about what is and is not news, while the last one relates to a very problem-atic area in organ donation: the unfairness of lavishing media attention on some cases and not on a whole host of others.

In September 1986, the Canadian federal health minister Jake Epp and his wife visited the Children's Hospital of Western Ontario in London, where they met a four-year-old Winnipeg boy who was awaiting a liver to replace his rapidly failing one. The young child happened to have been born on an Indian reserve in the politician's home riding of Provencher. The minister, in coop-eration with the director of the transplant program, decided to go public to plead this child's case, while other children quietly died of liver failure. This last point came under criticism, and the head of the transplant program responded, saying that he felt that he had to be an advocate for this child. No explanation was given for the fact that such advocacy is not in universal use.

FUTURE ISSUES YET UNRESOLVED

As discussions of the economics of medical care and the cost-effectiveness of many high-tech procedures begin to dominate the planning of North American health care, it becomes increas-ingly obvious that myriad problems are still unresolved. Trans-plantation is a significant problem area. Fundamental questions about whether this type of treatment should even be a part of our health care services are beginning to be raised more and more frequently. Many of those who work in the field see no rea-son to even ask the question, while others, who are looking at the larger picture, have more difficulty justifying the financial out-put for such a relatively small number of patients.

When the state of Oregon decided to take drastic measures in curbing its health care costs, while attempting to ensure at least basic care to all its citizens, it concluded that, while money for kidney transplants was well spent, bone marrow, heart, liver, and pancreas transplants would not be funded in order that more people would be covered for basic services. The governor was quoted as saying, 'How can we spend every nickel in sup-port of a few people when thousands never see a doctor or eat a decent meal?' (Balk 1990, 1129). His sentiments have been echoed by others: 'Is it appropriate for a relatively small number of people to benefit from public financing of an expensive technology when a larger number of people could benefit from expenditures on a broader range of less expensive health problems?' (Kutner 1987, 23).

While organ donation and transplantation have probably received more than their share of the media attention, many of the unanswered ethical questions never arise in this arena at all. These unresolved dilemmas will continue to plague transplanters, and it is in the best interest of both the medical personnel involved, and, more important, the patients, to deal with these problems as expeditiously as possible.

WHAT YOU CAN DO

Although relatively few of us will ever need an organ transplant, we are all being asked to consider organ donation. Just the other day, as I settled myself in an airplane seat, I noticed a slogan on a T-shirt worn by a young woman across the cabin. It said, 'Don't take your organs to heaven. Heaven knows who could use them here.' Clearly, this is one of the high-tech issues that we all need to consider.

- If you have not already signed an organ donor card, think about why you haven't done so yet. If you discover that you have no reason other than you have never thought about it, think about it and act. If you have concerns, write down your questions and then call your local transplant program, or liver, kidney, or heart foundation.
- If you decide that you can sign a card, talk to your family about it. Although your signed consent form is enough legally, transplant programs also seek consent of your family. They are the ones who will be left to deal with the decision.
- If you decide that signing a donor card is something you cannot do, discuss this with your family, help them to understand your point of view, and forget about it.

PART III

THE NEW EVERYDAY ETHICS

Some ethical challenges in medicine and health care have only recently become everyday concerns. They are, however, no less critical for everyone than those we presented in Part I. What makes them different is that they are growing in importance as time goes on and it is difficult to predict how they will develop.

The final five chapters will take you through some issues that you should be concerned about, if you are not already.

14

AIDS: Everyone's Concern

In the early 1980s, while the medical profession battled the fear-mongering that characterized media coverage of herpes infection, a new and even more deadly scourge was upon us that had yet to be discovered by either medical science or the media. By the early 1990s, we were faced with a whole host of fears and dilemmas surrounding HIV infection and AIDS. Although people feared herpes, they were terrified of AIDS. While herpes might paralyse your sex life, AIDS might take away your life – period. Now, while millions of dollars are being poured into research that might lead to treatment and cure of HIV infection, the medical profession is grappling with a growing number of moral questions about AIDS.

In early 1991, newspapers across North America were full of stories about an HIV-infected Florida dentist who had apparently passed the virus on to at least three of his patients. Prior to this time, it was widely believed that it was almost impossible for a health professional of any kind to transmit the virus if he or she followed the usual, recommended precautions. Now, the health professions had to stand up and publicly defend their unwritten policies regarding maintenance of the privacy of the individual health care worker.

At about the same time, researchers at the University of Toronto reported in the popular press the findings of a North American survey of doctors' attitudes towards telling patients about their own HIV status. Fully 75 per cent of the 254 doctors in the study revealed that they would refuse to tell their patients if they tested positive for the AIDS virus. At the same time, most doctors felt it was their right to know the HIV status of their patients. One of the researchers was quoted in the press as saying, 'In general, it appears that doctors seem to regard going off to the gulf war as a risk, but an acceptable risk, while caring for an HIV patient is not seen as an acceptable risk' (Taylor and Mickleburgh 1991).

Thus, it seems that AIDS is, indeed, everyone's concern, and for health professionals it is both a personal and a professional problem. We need to look closely at the ethical dimension of the medical problems that accompany what has been called the AIDS epidemic in North America. We also need to be comfortable with the direction of the answers that physicians are offering us.

WHAT WE KNOW ABOUT AIDS TODAY

There are two distinct areas of what we know about AIDS today and what you need to consider as you make a decision about the morality of how medical practitioners are dealing with it. First, there is objective information about HIV and the infection; second, there is the subjective response to the issue, in other words how we feel about it. Although the subjectivity of our feelings about HIV infection does not always reflect accurately the objective information, it is just as potent in its potential to cause problems.

First, let's deal with what we know about AIDS on an objective plane. An abundance of literature is available to the average person today from which to acquire objective information about AIDS. Practically every government and private organization that has any interest in health issues in general, or AIDS in particular, has produced some kind of informational brochure.

According to a Canadian federal government Health and Welfare brochure produced in 1990, this is what AIDS is: 'AIDS stands for Acquired Immunodeficiency Syndrome. AIDS is the advanced stage of the disease caused by the HIV- Human Immunodeficiency Virus. This virus attacks and seriously damages the

immune system, its defence against disease. Without this protection of the immune system, people with AIDS suffer from
fatal infections and cancer' (Health and Welfare Canada 1990).
The brochure goes on to say that Canada has one of the highest
rates of HIV infection among developed nations, estimating that
50,000 are already infected. No one is yet certain whether everyone who is infected with HIV will develop full-blown cases of
AIDS. However, recent studies that looked back on the course of
the disease in infected individuals estimate that 48 per cent of
those infected with the virus will develop AIDS after ten years
(Rachlis 1990).

As most consumers are aware, from mass-media coverage,
HIV is spread primarily through sexual contact, contaminated
needles, and blood products. Although widely believed to be a
disease of gay men when first identified, HIV infection and the
AIDS that follows, and results in death, are clearly diseases that
anyone can contract, given the right set of circumstances. Casual
contact with a person infected with HIV is not one of those circumstances. But it is misunderstanding of this issue – how the
virus is spread – that leads us into some of the subjectivity of
what we know about this devastating disease today.

Another area of concern has been the risk of acquiring HIV
from an infected health professional, and vice versa. Following
the case of the Florida dentist, the U.S. Centers for Disease Control (CDC) reviewed the validity of their previous recommenda-
tions for the types of precautions that health professionals
should take to protect both themselves and their patients. They
estimated that the risk of a doctor or other health professional
contracting the virus from a patient to be relatively small, at
about 0.3 per cent, and the risk in the other direction, a patient
contracting the disease from a health professional, to be even
smaller (Steben 1992). The CDC indicates that mandatory HIV
testing of health professionals is unnecessary.

AIDS, however, is more than a physiological disease process
that can be defined by its 'natural history,' as doctors call it; it
has become an extraordinarily complex social issue whose
dilemmas have polarized the population. How people feel about

AIDS and, the people who are affected by the virus, and what
they believe as a result of those feelings, are at the root of many
of the ethical problems we face on the AIDS front. In addition,
the feelings of health professionals and of health care consumers
about AIDS are not always the same.

HOW DOCTORS FEEL ABOUT AIDS

While we recognize the dangers of generalizing about how a
group feels about any issue, we can probably make a case that, in
general, doctors have two different feelings about HIV infection.
The first relates to infected patients and the second to infected
physicians or other health professionals.

As mentioned earlier, in 1990, the mass media carried the
results of a study conducted by a behavioural scientist who discovered that most doctors would not tell their patients if they
themselves carried HIV. Even more disturbing than this, perhaps, was the attitude of the more than 500 medical students,
the doctors of tomorrow, who also participated in the study. The
medical students were found to have what was described as an
exaggerated fear of contracting AIDS. Here are some of the specific findings as reported in the press:

- 70 per cent have a negative view of homosexuals;
- 50 per cent would have concerns about sharing their facilities
  with an AIDS clinic;
- almost 50 per cent believe that medical students should have
  the right to refuse to treat patients carrying HIV (Canadian
  Press 1990)

One of the most distressing findings is that, despite current
medical knowledge that HIV cannot be transmitted by casual
contact, one in six medical students still say that they would not
leave their child in a class with an HIV-infected student. The
researcher was quoted in the press as saying, 'One response to
this survey is to say all these students are insensitive, prejudiced
jerks, but that isn't very productive' (Canadian Press 1990). Fur-

ther findings, however, also indicated that more than 80 per cent of the students did say that they would, indeed, accept HIV-infected individuals as patients and that they would like more information about the issues involved in caring for these patients.

In general, the negative attitudes towards AIDS that have often been found among doctors have been linked to what is widely believed to be a particular fear of death the people in the medical profession seem to possess (Solomon and Mead 1987). As two researchers in the San Francisco Biopsychosocial AIDS Project have said: 'AIDS is doubly threatening to the physician. He or she may be "used to" death and dying , but will find unsettling a fatal disease, among generally healthy young patients, for which there is no effective treatment. His or her sense of invulnerability and of competence are both threatened' (Solomon and Mead 1987, 13)

PUBLIC OPINION ABOUT AIDS

While the attitudes of physicians towards AIDS in both themselves and their patients may cause problems in practice, the attitudes of the general public only compound them. Fear is the best way to describe how people feel.

This fear was illustrated recently in Britain when it became publicly known that a number of doctors who had AIDS continued to practise. The first case was that of a Dr Shuttleworth, an obstetrician-gynaecologist, who had tested HIV positive after a ten-year career that involved treating about 17,000 women and operating on 6,000 of them. This case triggered a number of announcements of other doctors and a midwife who had either tested positive for HIV or died of AIDS.

The Shuttleworth case resulted in more than 10,000 telephone calls to the local health authorities over a two-day period. During this same two-day period, 374 of his former patients underwent HIV testing (Lord 1993). While this resulted in calls for mandatory HIV testing of health professionals, it was pointed out that there is only one documented case of a health professional infecting patients with HIV, while there are 150 alleged cases of patients infecting doctors.

Although people seem to fear HIV infection and AIDS when forced to confront the issue directly, it seems that the average middle-class North American still feels quite distanced from the so-called epidemic. Despite recent media attention to the fact that AIDS does not discriminate, there is still a feeling that it is something that happens to gay men, drug abusers, the sexually promiscuous, and the occasional unfortunate blood recipient.

MANDATORY TESTING?

The fact that doctors and other health professionals are at a greater risk of contracting HIV from patients than vice versa has resulted in some physicians and other health professionals coming forward to demand mandatory testing of patients and the provision of test results to any involved caregiver. This proposition has received mixed reactions from the medical profession, and outright condemnation from AIDS activist groups.

According to article 8 of the Canadian Medical Association's Code of Ethics (1990), physicians are to 'recommend only diagnostic procedures that are believed necessary to assist in the care of the patient ...,' which effectively precludes blood testing for the purposes of protecting the caregiver. In a letter to the *Canadian Medical Association Journal,* which had previously published an article on this issue that provoked considerable response, one doctor indicated that, while in general he agreed with clause 8 of the code of ethics, he felt that the AIDS situation is different. He believes that the significance of the AIDS threat could never have been contemplated when such codes were developed. He said: 'most of us are not suicidal, and we entered our profession believing that we still had the right to protect our lives and those of our loved ones. Taking a blind risk that may endanger human lives – mine, those of my spouse and my unborn child, and those of other patients – is not my idea of ethics' (Lambert 1992, 577).

AIDS activist groups, on the other hand, believe that having the HIV status of every patient available to health care workers is not likely to reduce transmission. It is likely to result in less care being made available for AIDS sufferers. They believe that, when the recommended universal precautions are taken to prevent transmission of infectious diseases, health care workers are not at significantly enough risk to warrant divulging this kind of information about patients. Furthermore, they believe that making this kind of testing mandatory is likely to make people who are at risk avoid any contact with caregivers so as not to be tested.

It is fear on the parts of both doctors and health care consumers that places obstacles in the way of rational, clear-headed decision making when faced with the many moral dilemmas sparked by AIDS.

THE UNANSWERED MORAL QUESTIONS

Physicians generally try to work from the following three commitments:

- to give the best care that they can;
- to be honest;
- to be trustworthy (Parsons and Parsons 1990).

These commitments are tried mightily when physicians must deal with the unresolved questions that arise from the AIDS issue. Here are several of the basic questions.

1. *What are the limits of patient confidentiality when the patient is infected with HIV?*
While physicians will often fight almost to the death to protect the privacy of the doctor–patient relationship in theory, AIDS is one of those issues that causes doctors to face an increasing need for others to know about the patient's condition. Ideally, if a doctor is trustworthy, he or she will not break a patient's confidence. When AIDS is involved, the situation is less than ideal.

When an HIV-positive bisexual, married man refuses to tell

his wife of his affliction, where are the limits of the physician's responsibility to keep the secret? Should he or she respect the patient's wishes not to divulge this information because of the social implications, or should the doctor tell the spouse to protect her and her children? A Canadian Medical Association discussion paper published in 1989 had this to say about answering this question:

As a general principle, physicians must respect patients' rights to privacy and confidentiality ...

Physicians have an obligation to ensure that contact tracing takes place with respect to identified or readily identifiable persons at risk of HIV transmission who would not otherwise be aware that they were at such risk. (Gilmore and Somerville 1989, 22, 24)

This guideline for physicians from CMA is still a bit unclear.

On one hand, doctors with AIDS patients are told that they have an obligation to maintain patient confidentiality. On the other hand, they are told that they have an obligation to trace contacts, but this stipulation is phrased in such a way that they would still be unsure about the solidity of their ethical ground. The bureaucratic doublespeak goes like this: 'Such compulsory contact tracing is only ethically justifiable if it is the least invasive, least restrictive, reasonably available and likely to be effective means of informing' people who would not otherwise be aware of their risk (Gilmore and Somerville 1989, 24). With guidelines like these, it is no surprise that physicians have extreme difficulty making a decision with which they feel comfortable and which will be acceptable to health care consumers.

2. *Is it ethical for a doctor to refuse to treat a person with HIV?*
While, in general, doctors believe in the obligation to treat, we have already established that they retain the right to refuse to treat anyone for any reason, unless in an emergency situation. Given the fear that many doctors seem to have of HIV infection, it might be reasonable to assume that this right could result in a

dearth of physicians available to treat those who desperately need them.

In general, if a doctor has a moral objection to treating a particular patient, as in the case of abortion, then the refusal is justified. If, on the other hand, the refusal is based on fear, the reason is not a good one. People who choose to be doctors are exposed to considerably more health hazards in an average day than are most other people, and they know this from the outset of their training.

On an average day, a family physician might be exposed to influenza, chicken pox, meningitis, strep throat, hepatitis ... the list goes on. The results of studies on the risk of a health professional contracting AIDS have concluded that the risk is too small to justify refusal to treat, and that the risk of contracting hepatitis is twenty to thirty times greater (Grady 1989). The Canadian Medical Association discussion paper indicates that 'unreasonable refusals to care for patients with HIV/AIDS are ethically unacceptable' (Gilmore and Somerville 1989, 30).

Historically, there have always been doctors who fled their patients in the face of risk to their own health. During the plague years in Europe, doctors who feared for their health deserted their patients but, as has been the tradition of medical practitioners for centuries, these doctors were denounced by their colleagues (Kluge 1991).

3. *When the rights of a doctor or a doctor's obligations conflict with the rights of an individual patient, whose rights should take precedence?*
This is a very good example of a typical ethical dilemma whose solution will necessarily be harmful to someone. One of the parties involved will be harmed regardless of what action is taken.

The usual problems here stem from two situations:

- when the doctor has to balance the individual's right to privacy with the public's right to be protected; and
- when the doctor's right to privacy has to be balanced against the patient's right to know.

In a study reported in the *Journal of the American Medical Association* in 1989, researchers asked a U.S. nation-wide sample of people what they thought about doctors and HIV. Eighty per cent of the people in the study said that they believed that doctors should inform their patients of their HIV status, regardless of their specialty. In addition, 45 per cent said that those who are HIV positive should not be practising medicine at all. While most people seem to recognize the situations when they are in the greatest risk, the researchers referred to this paradox: 'the public's desire to avoid people with HIV disease seems much stronger than their perception of risk of transmission would "rationally" predict' (Gerbert and colleagues 1989, 1971). Thus, it seems that even if, intellectually, consumers realize that they are at extremely low risk of contracting HIV from their doctors, the fear persists. The doctor's right to privacy is in direct conflict with the patient's right to be informed of *all* the risks associated with treatment – in this case with the person giving the treatment.

The best that can be said at the present time is that health professionals who are HIV positive and who engage in activities that are invasive in nature, such as surgery, have been told that they are to restrict those activities. In addition, the guidelines from the Centers for Disease Control specify the precautions that should be taken by every health professional to protect both the caregiver and the patient. The American Medical Association, however, has stated that any amount of risk to a patient is too much risk. Since three to six months may pass before a person infected tests positive for HIV, even regular, routine testing of all health care workers would not achieve zero risk for patients.

This guideline of zero risk is also problematic for the medical profession. 'There is a paradox in demanding that physicians provide care for the patient with a particular disease, but if the physician contracts the disease, also demanding that the physician be excluded from the profession' (Dickey 1989, 2002). This paradox has made both physicians and their patients unhappy with the guidelines currently available.

4. *Is it morally acceptable to spend more money on AIDS than on other diseases that affect and kill more people?*

This is a fundamental question of how to allocate scarce resources. These resources include not only money, but also laboratory space, time, and highly trained researchers. In 1992, $1.3 billion was spent in the United States on AIDS, millions more than was spent on heart disease during the same period (Gray 1993). At first glance, this might seem like an unusually lopsided situation. If we consider that, at the present time, more people die of heart disease than AIDS, the allocation of resources doesn't seem to make sense. What we really need, then, is to be able to determine how many people are likely to be affected by HIV in the future if we don't spend money on researching it today.

AIDS today has been compared with leprosy in antiquity. There have even been suggestions that those so afflicted should be quarantined. The bottom line in any discussion of the medical profession's ethical approach to AIDS and HIV infection is that there are few good answers available at the present time. These issues are so complex today that lack of real understanding of the disease and the fear that accompanies not knowing only serve to complicate things further. It is the responsibility of each of us to be informed at least about the currently available facts to protect ourselves physically and to help the medical profession to make some difficult decisions.

15

Forbidden Sex:
Sexual Abuse of Patients by Doctors

Even Hippocrates had thought about it when he wrote, 'Whatever house I enter, I will go therein for the benefit of the sick and I will stand free from any voluntary criminal action and corrupt deed and the seduction of females or males, be they slaves or free.' As we flash forward two thousand years, we come to the 1990s, where the phrase 'sex in the forbidden zone' (Rutter 1986) is making an all-too-common appearance in the mass media as doctors are taken to task for engaging in sexual relationships with their patients. At first glance, this may seem to the lesser informed to be a matter less of professional ethics than of personal choice. By most current definitions, however, this behaviour does, indeed, pose serious moral problems for modern doctors.

From the perspective of the involved physician, American psychiatrist Dr Peter Rutter first described this concern as the allure of the forbidden when he defined the phrase as meaning 'any sexual contact that occurred within the professional relationships of trust' (1986, 11). From the perspective of the popular media, at least, it is one of the hottest ethical problems in the medical profession today. As a consequence, sexual abuse of patients, as the medical profession defines it, is currently among the highest-profile moral dilemmas faced by doctors. How organized medicine is dealing with this problem is the focus of our discussion. As one writer in the medical press wrote recently, 'Having erotic feelings for a patient is normal, but surrendering to those feelings is not ...' (Lowry 1993, 27).

The bottom line, from an ethical perspective, then, is that doctors are not supposed to engage in any level of sexual activity with patients. Centuries ago Hippocrates perceived this; today's medical professionals recognize this too.

POWER: INEQUALITY SPAWNS PROBLEMS

As we discussed earlier in this book, there is an inherent inequality in the relationship between doctor and patient. Although this situation has changed somewhat with the advent of the health-consumerist movement and the better-informed patient, it still remains a fact: in the therapeutic relationship, the caregiver is in a greater power position than is the person to whom the care is given. Knowledge and control are at the heart of the inequality, and inequality spawns the ethical dilemma.

In the past five years, doctors have begun to examine this problem of sexual indiscretion as worthy of serious consideration. As one medical board report says: 'sexual abuse of patients by physicians represents a serious abuse of power and as such, compromises a physician's ability to deliver competent medical care ... Where an established physician/patient relationship exists there are no circumstances where sexual activity between a physician and his/her patient is appropriate' ('Report on sexual abuse', 1992). Clearly, as a group, physicians recognize this problem in their ranks. What they are doing about it is worthy of our consideration.

THE SERIOUSNESS OF THE PROBLEM

Reading the newspapers today might lead one to conclude that all physicians are not to be trusted. Any time we enter a doctor's examining-room, we should be wary. This, of course, breaks down the trust that is necessary for a good relationship with one's doctor.

Some of the studies of physicians' involvement with patients estimate that 10 per cent of male doctors and 2 per cent of female doctors are guilty of sexual abuse of patients. In half of these situations, the abuse consists of actual sexual intercourse. In the other half, the abuse can range from calling a female patient 'honey' to sexual touching. Many women wouldn't consider their doctor's use of a term of endearment such as 'honey' grounds for alleging sexual abuse, nor would most doctors have intended it to be; however, there have been instances when such familiarity has been perceived to be abusive. There is, of course, some difficulty in obtaining accurate statistics to reflect the problem as there is a tendency to rely on self-reported behaviour in surveys of doctors.

DEFINING THE BOUNDARIES OF THE ACCEPTABLE

While it is generally considered acceptable for two consenting adults to enter into any kind of relationship that they choose, where doctors are concerned a consenting patient is no different, from an ethical perspective, than one who did not consent. Under any circumstances such a relationship is inappropriate, and the physician is to blame, since, by its very nature, this unequal relationship places the patient in a position of vulnerability and the doctor in the position of abusing his or her position of power. In theory, patients are not really able to consent freely in these relationships because they are characteristically exploitive. This being the case, we need to define what behaviour is considered to be appropriate and what is not.

Consider the following: Sharon Connors, a twenty-seven-year-old, has just entered her doctor's office for her annual pap smear. She has been going to this same male doctor for the past ten years and, in fact, he performed her first internal examination when she came to him at age seventeen for a prescription for birth control pills. He has already seen her through an early marriage and an unpleasant divorce.

As she enters the examining-room, he places his hand on her shoulder and says, 'How are you doing today, Sharon?'

She smiles, and they engage in small talk for a few minutes before he leaves so that she may ready herself for the examination. When he returns, they continue their familiar banter.

As he prepares to conduct the examination he says, 'Could you move your bottom down a couple of inches, honey?' She does so, and the examination progresses. Sharon leaves happy as usual with her treatment from her trusted family doctor. However, some questions have been raised by such an encounter:

- Should the doctor have touched Sharon's arm outside of the physical examination?
- Was it proper for the doctor to refer to Sharon as 'honey'?
- Does Sharon have a case for sexual misconduct against her doctor?

In answer to the last question, Sharon probably never even thought about the appropriateness of her doctor's behaviour. She likes his approach and feels comfortable with it. Other patients, however, may not feel the same way. In fact, these very issues are some of the grounds for complaints against doctors, whether they are justified or not. Are there any clear guidelines, then, about what does and what does not constitute sexual misconduct?

While patients are having trouble defining these boundaries, individual doctors, as well as their professional associations, are also having difficulty. These are some of the behaviours that have been deemed to constitute sexual misconduct (or 'sexual violation,' 'sexual impropriety,' or 'sexual abuse') on the part of a physician:

- sexual intercourse with a patient
- inappropriate touching, including touching the genitals without gloves
- making comments with sexual overtones
- requesting dates
- watching patients undress
- subjecting patients to examinations with medical students present without their expressed consent
- criticizing a patient's sexual orientation

As you can see, some of these are somewhat subjective, to say the least. Is calling a patient 'honey' considered to have sexual overtones? Some patients think so; others do not. The result is that doctors are having a great deal of trouble determining what is appropriate behaviour, and this is even having an impact on their medical care. One physician related a story about his own wife's gynaecologist. His wife informed him that her doctor had stopped doing breast examinations because of his fear that he might be accused of violating his patients (Lowry 1993). This kind of backlash is extremely dangerous.

Adult patients generally know when their doctor has overstepped the boundary of the appropriate because of how a particular kind of behaviour makes them feel. On the other hand, it seems to be more difficult for the physicians to decide how to act with patients since an innocent, off-the-cuff remark to one patient may be acceptable in that patient's eyes, but unacceptable in another's. How, then, can doctors make this distinction?

One suggestion that has been made to doctors is that they first must be aware of the warning signs that are evidently there. For example, talking to patients about their own personal problems, vulnerabilities, and marital difficulties indicates that they are entering into the forbidden zone (Moore 1992).

HOW TO DEAL WITH THE PROBLEM

In a number of jurisdictions, laws to protect patients from abuse by their doctors have been proposed and passed. Most entail some type of mandatory reporting by colleagues, if appropriate. It will be some time before the effects of these laws can be evaluated.

What, then, as a patient, should you expect from your doctor? The short answer is: respect. Although a clear definition of respectful behaviour is difficult to develop, here are some of the more concrete ways doctors have been advised to reduce the perception of sexual impropriety. This is what you should expect:

- A doctor should respect your right to privacy before, during, and after your medical examination. You should be left alone to prepare, unless you need help, in which case a female care-giver should be available to female patients. You should be adequately draped during the examination, and you should be afforded privacy to redress afterwards.
- A doctor should prepare you for any physical examinations by explaining what he or she will be doing before beginning.
- A doctor should limit his or her questions about your sexual history to those necessary for your immediate care. In the age of AIDS, it is increasingly common for questions about sexual partners to be asked before an internal examination. This is to be expected.
- Male doctors should ensure that a female staff member is present during internal and breast examinations on female patients. Some patients, however, are uncomfortable having another person present during an examination. If you are one of these people, you will have to discuss this with your doctor. Under current circumstances, he may insist. (At the present time, there has been little call for the presence of another male when a female doctor is performing a genital examination, but if a male patient requests one, the doctor should be expected to respect it.)
- Doctors should not make tasteless or vulgar remarks or jokes, or casually touch patients in ways that could be interpreted as suggestive.
- Doctors should not engage patients in conversation about their own problems, especially sexual or marital concerns.
- Doctors should not ask their patients for dates.

If you feel uncomfortable about your physician's style or language, you should inform him or her. Given all of these restrictions, one is reminded of the doctor who chooses to practise in an underserviced area where all of the population within miles are patients. What kind of a social life does this doctor have in his own community? Evidently, he or she has none.

16

When They Tell You You're Too Old

When the turn-of-the-decade issues of magazines began rolling off the presses at the end of December 1989 to assess the past and predict the future, *Newsweek*'s special issue ignored the economy and technology and focused instead on people – who we are and who we are becoming. They called their article about the ageing of the North American population 'The Geezer Boom.' While failing to offer a flattering picture of the ageing population, the headline did point to the inevitability of the baby boomers moving into middle age and beyond.

Unflattering descriptions of older adults abound in a society that has been obsessed with youth for so long, and medicine is not immune. When physician-author Samuel Shem wrote about them in his novel *The House of God*, he called them 'GOMERs,' which he said stood for 'Get Out Of My Emergency Room,' a term that is a part of the hospital folk language of many an intern and resident in many teaching hospitals across the continent (George and Dundes 1978). Although the actual origin of the term is unknown, it is used to refer to 'an unkempt, unsavory, chronic problem patient' (George and Dundes 1978, 572). As disrespectful as the term is, its use can be examined for what it represents to modern medicine. The ageing individual is getting closer to death every day, and it is death that seems to be the enemy to the modern doctor. It hardly seems odd, then, for doctors-in-training to make jokes about what they fear. They are, after all, only human.

While the ethical problems that relate to physicians and older adults are really not very different from the general kinds of dilemmas that we have been discussing, some special circumstances surround the problems in this context. In light of the fact that the bulge of the North American public is fast approaching older adulthood, some of the dilemmas are likely to become even more problematic as time goes on.

We'll examine the general problem of ageism in North American society, what modern medicine has done and not done for ageing people, and whether or not the medical profession has been any more successful in dealing with the moral dilemmas surrounding the elderly than with those related to other times in life.

AGEISM IN NORTH AMERICA

It does not take very sophisticated mathematics to determine that, by the year 2030, the last of the baby boomers will be senior citizens. This means that a third of the population will be the aged. Given the prevalence of the aged in society by that time, you might think that our attitudes towards older adults are likely to have changed dramatically by then. If so, the changes will have to be enormous.

Ageism has been compared to racism. People make assumptions about the capabilities and potential contributions of individuals based on their chronological age, and the problem has been rampant for some time. Under increasing scrutiny for the past few years, the practice of mandatory retirement has been given as an example of blatant discrimination based on age. Despite the possible wisdom of the idea that older people who have had their chance at life ought to make way so that younger people might have more opportunities, the idea that age on its own is a determinant of capabilities is fast becoming a dinosaur. Attitudes of some people, however, are slow to change.

If you are not old, it is difficult to imagine what it will be like, and once you are there, you can't go back. Or can you? In 1979, a twenty-six-year-old industrial engineer decided that she wanted to find out. Using make-up and specially constructed prosthetics, Pat Moore transformed herself into an eighty-eight-year-old woman and embarked upon a two-year journey that took her to 116 cities in 14 U.S. states and 2 Canadian provinces. What she discovered is bone-chilling to anyone looking down the road towards old age.

To say that her experience was not pleasant would be an understatement. At the best of times, she was ignored; at the worst, physically beaten. But she found that, among older people, she was welcomed and treated with compassion and brotherhood. Still, the experience, retold in her book *Disguised: A True Story*, published in 1985, tells us that the respect that was offered our elders in earlier years seems to be all but forgotten in modern society.

In medical care today, the issue of discrimination based on age takes on a slightly different complexion. Consider the problems faced by a transplant program in trying to make decisions about the best recipient for an organ, a scarce resource, as we have already established. For a long time, discrimination on the grounds of age was firmly established in organ-procurement agencies across the continent. This was a medical decision that was based on the unsubstantiated assumption that transplantation in older patients would not be as likely to have a successful outcome. Thus, it seemed only prudent to use such a scarce resource as organs on a person for whom the success of the procedure was more likely. Further research resulted in the rejection of that assumption. When faced with two worthy recipients, both of whom have predictably similar medical responses, the reason for passing over the older of them today is often simply age.

Another reason why the issue of age-related discrimination is a very important dilemma is the sheer numbers of older people who are likely to need the services of doctors and hospitals in the future. As we age, our bodies deteriorate and we tend to come in contact with the health care system more frequently. As two writers have said, 'On average, people over the age of 65 years suffer from between three and four chronic disorders. The likelihood of hospitalization in any given year is 18 per cent' (Jahnigen and Schrier 1986, 457). How the elderly are treated by the medical profession, then, is very important in any discussion of modern medical ethics.

WHAT MODERN MEDICINE HAS DONE FOR AGEING

For the past couple of decades, the North American public has been obsessed with youth. This obsession has encompassed how we think about our looks, our careers, our lives, and, most important, our health. We are interested in longevity and in being as healthy as possible.

Since the turn of the century, the average life span for a North American has increased by about twenty-eight years. This is largely the result of modern medicine. While medicine could treat illness in 1900, it could not cure it. Thanks to the advent of antibiotics, the toll taken by infectious diseases on large numbers of young people and children early in the century is now purely a matter of history. And the advances of the past two decades have resulted in phenomenal abilities to treat and cure a wide variety of acute diseases that have afflicted mankind for years. There has been little improvement, however, in the long-term treatment and cure of the chronic diseases and, now that we all live longer, we can expect to suffer from three or four of those chronic diseases as we approach the end of life.

How long could human beings live if there were no disease? Would our bodies last forever? Scientists who have made careers out of trying to answer this question say no, our bodies would not last forever, and have argued that the human life span is biologically fixed, at about 110–15 years (Lusky 1986). Realistically, however, since no society is likely to rid itself completely of disease or accidents causing death and disability, human life expectancy is, on average, likely to level out at about 85 years, close to its current level.

When we talk about the chronic diseases that we now live long enough to acquire, we are talking about a specific list. A study reported in 1986 indicated that the following ten diseases are the ones most likely to befall us:

1. cardiovascular disease (diseases of the heart and blood vessels such as high blood pressure, heart attacks, and strokes)
2. musculoskeletal diseases (those affecting the bones and muscles, such as arthritis and osteoporosis)
3. hearing problems
4. vision problems
5. nutritional problems (poor nutritional habits)
6. endocrine disorders (diabetes)
7. gastrointestinal diseases (diseases such as lactose intolerance, bowel cancer, diverticulosis)
8. allergic conditions
9. respiratory diseases (chronic obstructive lung disease, emphysema, lung cancer)
10. dermatologic conditions (skin cancer and premalignant conditions, dry itchy skin) (Lusky 1986).

Thus, the first legacy of modern medical technology to ageing patients is a longer life with, perhaps, more chronic illness, and the second, which naturally flows from the first, is the dilemma of quantity versus quality of life.

As physicians have acquired the ability to cheat death, a new twist on an old problem has arisen. That problem is the ever-increasing difficulty of knowing when to stop treating. Dr Nancy Jecker of the University of Washington has said this about knowing when to stop: 'only the physician who understands natural limits and uses this understanding to set wise boundaries avoids the error of excessive confidence' (1991). The implication here, then, is that a doctor who refuses to recognize when the time has come to stop treating does not know either the limits of modern medicine or his or her own limits.

Clearly, as patients age, and death comes ever closer, there is a tendency for those doctors trained in modern warfare against the enemy death to try everything humanly possible. Sometimes, in an effort to delay the inevitable as long as possible, they even try the impossible. The patient, if he or she is able, and his or her family must play a part in helping these doctors to reach a decision to stop treatment. They can reassure them that it is 'all right' to do so.

Hippocrates could never have foreseen the technological marvels that have been developed in the past two decades, but as long ago as the 5th century B.C., physicians of the Hippocratic tradition saw that they needed to be aware of the limitations of their art, and to know when to stop.

One other effect of modern medicine is worth our consideration before we look at specific ethical dilemmas that surround the care of ageing patients. As we mentioned earlier, in the chapter on the intensive care unit, this is what one author has called the development of a new kind of patient, the 'high-tech chronic' (Hutchison 1988). These are the often older patients for whom medical technology offers but a slim hope of quality of life, but for whom it is tried anyway. These are patients who are nearing the end of their natural lives and are resuscitated, for example, only to require long-term care of an intense, technologically oriented nature. The rise in the number of these patients is sometimes the result of the inability of some members of the medical profession to know when to stop. In fairness, however, doctors are not entirely to blame. As consumers have gained a little knowledge about a lot of things through the mass media, they have played an ever-increasing role in health care decisions. While this is a good thing generally sometimes it leads family members to exert pressure on health care professionals to try anything possible, even in the face of medical futility. Fear of repercussions such as litigation, as we have already discussed, causes doctors to follow those wishes from time to time, with poor outcomes.

SPECIFIC ETHICAL DILEMMAS RELATED TO AGEING

There are three general questions in relation to ageing that modern medicine and its consumers need to examine. All too often these issues are regarded as equal across the lifespan, but we contend that they are not. Some problems become exaggerated as the patients age.

1. *Are older adults accorded the same consideration regarding their right to self-determination? In other words, do doctors let their older patients be autonomous?*

We have already discussed the problems that the medical profession has had for many years in letting patients become partners in health care, and consumers have helped the medical profession to take great strides in this direction. The partnership model is not, however, universal, nor is the right accorded to everyone equally. Consider what happens when an older patient is diagnosed with terminal cancer. If the family is close by, the patient's daughter, for example, is as likely to be consulted as is the patient herself. In addition, doctors and families have even gone so far as to make decisions about whether or not older patients should even be told their diagnoses. This lingering paternalism in medical care is then adopted by the family as well, and all of them begin to treat the older person as if he or she were a child, no longer capable of having a useful say in decisions.

Another issue here is that physicians often seem to have difficulty accepting the decisions made by older adults. There is an undercurrent of feeling that even a minimal amount of mental incapacity renders the older person unable to take an active part in decision making.

Finally, many older adults today feel more comfortable leaving the decision making to their doctors. They were brought up with a very different attitude towards the medical profession than the baby boomers have been. Difficulties can arise, however, when the baby-boomer child fails to understand that Mother or Father might be more comfortable taking a lesser role in decision making.

2. *Are older patients accorded the same level of confidentiality in their encounters with their physicians?*

The answer to this question is a direct consequence of the lack of autonomy given to older people within the health care system. When a patient's son, daughter, or spouse is consulted about a treatment decision, the patient's privacy is often being invaded. While a doctor would never consider discussing a young husband's personal medical condition with his wife without his permission, that same doctor may not think twice about giving test results over the phone to the spouse of an older patient without consent. This invasion of privacy is often done under the guise of care for the individual, doing what is best for him or her, but the result is that the confidentiality of the encounter between doctor and patient is seen as somehow different when the patient is older.

3. *Should older people be given the same consideration as younger people in the allocation of scarce resources?*
This is an especially difficult decision, and the behaviour of the medical profession in this area is often a reflection of the difficulty that society in general has in letting go and making way for others. In the best of all possible worlds, where everyone is concerned about the greater good, this would likely not be a problem at all. Whatever is in the best interests of society at large would be acceptable to everyone (if we could come to a consensus on what is, indeed, in the best interests of society). Sometimes that might mean passing the older patient by, and sometimes it might mean placing that person first in line.

THE ETHICAL PHYSICIAN FOR THE OLDER ADULT

For many years, you may have had the happy experience of developing a trusting relationship with a family physician. If this person has been one of your contemporaries, as you approach retirement, so too will your doctor. This is a problem for many older adults. It is one thing to assess the ethical approach of a doctor you know well and trust anyway, but quite another to do the same with a health professional you hardly know at all. It is less the substance of what a doctor learned in medical school than it is a matter of personal values when it comes to the issue of whether this doctor's value system is congruent with yours.

Before we look at who might be the best doctor for an older adult, we need to keep in mind one other thing. As we have said before, doctors are only human and, as such, they have their foibles, their prejudices, and their preferences. A doctor who enjoys delivering babies and caring for young families may not receive as much fulfilment from caring for older adults.

Who, then, is a suitably ethical doctor for an older adult? These are some of the questions of importance to ageing patients that need to be discussed with doctors:

- Does the doctor share your attitudes about quality versus quantity of life?
- Does the doctor treat you with the level of respect with which you feel comfortable?
- Does the doctor patiently answer any and all questions that you have about your health care?
- Does the doctor treat you as the primary focus of the care and the decisions?
- Does the doctor stay actively involved in your care, even when you are referred to a specialist/consultant?
- Does the doctor consult you before revealing any medical information about you to your family?

While these may seem like simple things that we all take for granted, they are not so simple when they are overlooked, even when supposedly in the best interests of the patient.

Ethical treatment of older people is likely to become a high-profile issue as the North American age wave bulges towards new heights. Baby boomers have never been a complacent bunch and are not likely to be the same kind of health consumers as were their parents and grandparents. These issues are likely to become more contentious before they are solved to the satisfaction of doctors and consumers alike.

17
Death, Dying, and Doctors' Ethics

It has often been said, and even supported in a few studies, that people who choose medicine as a career have an unusually intense fear of death. Judging from the efforts to which many practitioners of modern medicine go to prevent this inevitable event, it seems, at least anecdotally, that this is the case. Those who have spent any time observing the health care system from within all have stories to tell that support this theory. Perhaps, from the point of view of the patient, under most circumstances this is a good thing. After all, if your life is in danger, don't you want a doctor who will do everything humanly possible to save it? The answer to that question should be a qualified 'sometimes,' and this is the basis for our discussion of modern doctors and their approach to death.

If there is one universal truth in life it is this: we are all going to die some day. Neither modern medical technology nor the most brilliant doctor in the world can prevent this. What these two can do together is make dying more comfortable both physically and emotionally, and postpone death, but that is, in the end, all they can do. Sometimes this is a very good thing. What doctors can forget is that a futile attempt to prevent death might just be the worst possible thing that has ever happened in a particular person's life.

Among the most sensitive ethical issues that face modern physicians are those that deal with concerns at the end of our lives. Now that it is possible to control the time of death to a degree, there have arisen the inevitable questions about who has the right to play God.

In addition to the dilemmas that relate to who can and should make these decisions, there is another, perhaps even more pervasive, moral problem surrounding dying in modern health care. This is the increasingly difficult problem of dealing with what we are calling the 'high-tech death.' As our ability to control life and death has evolved, modern health care facilities and their policies and procedures have all but removed humanity from this very universally human event. Today's death is, without doubt, technology-driven.

DEFINING THE MODERN DEATH

What is death? This might seem like an odd question to have to ask but, in light of modern health care, it begs to be answered. Obviously death means being no longer alive. With modern medical intervention, however, neither defining death nor defining what it means to be 'alive' is easy.

For centuries, death was an accepted part of human life, a passage that was inevitable and one to prepare for and take with loved ones close by, if at all possible. This is still the case in many less 'developed' cultures in the world today. Even as recently as the beginning of this century, most people in North America died at home. The bone-chilling fear of death that seems to have developed in North American society, coupled with the marvels of modern medicine, has moved death from the human event it once was to a medical event with the individual surrounded, not by loving family, but by flashing, beeping, and hissing machinery and white-coated strangers. The idea of having a 'dignified death,' if any death can be considered dignified, is a modern invention in response to this apparent loss of dignity.

If you die at home, your death is likely to be more personal and less medical. The fact is, however, that between 75 and 80 per cent of all deaths that occur on this continent occur in hospitals. Since there is such a high probability that you will, indeed, die in a hospital, you might want to sit up and take notice of how decisions about your life and death are likely to be made.

THE MODERN, HIGH-TECH DEATH

Before we finish examining what death means in modern medical practice, we need to define *cardiac arrest*. This definition will put the discussion of a hospital death in perspective.

We've all seen it on television. Every doctor show that has ever made it to prime time has had them on a regular basis. Often referred to by such euphemisms as a 'code' or an 'arrest,' a cardiac arrest is one of the most dramatic medical emergencies outside the operating room in a modern acute-care hospital. The nurse (it is most often a nurse) discovers the patient is not breathing. She or he quickly checks for a carotid pulse (the one in the neck that you use to check your heart rate during aerobic class), while reaching for the call bell and summoning help. A call is made to the 'arrest team,' whose pagers start beeping all around the hospital, and they begin their breathless arrivals within minutes. While waiting, the nurse begins cardiopulmonary resuscitation (CPR), using mouth-to-mouth breathing (or mouth-to-airway in this day of AIDS, if an airway is handy) and chest compression. Finally, someone takes over this exhausting job, and everyone falls into his or her routine function: the resident passes a breathing tube down into the lungs; the respiratory technologist begins 'bagging' (using a bag to blow air into the lungs); the intern starts an IV so that they will be able to 'push' the drugs that will follow; the resident barks out orders; the nurse places the electrodes on the patient's chest so that the heart beat may be monitored, draws up the medications, and charges the defibrillator; the resident call for everyone to 'clear' and they all stand back so he or she can administer an electrical shock designed to restart the fibrillating heart. If all of this doesn't work, they continue with the medications and repeat the procedures. At some point, a decision is made to stop, and the patient is allowed to continue being dead.

So, the short definition of a cardiac arrest is 'when an individual stops breathing and his or her heart stops beating.' Before the advent of CPR, this was otherwise known as 'death.' Since this is no longer the case, death, by definition, must be something different. But what is it?

The fact is, a person's brain doesn't actually die until almost ten minutes after the heart stops beating, but damage to it begins within three to four minutes without blood circulation. Thus, we have a new definition of death, and the new term 'brain death,' to which we referred in our discussion of organ donation.

Now that we all know what death is and is not in the modern hospital, we can begin to examine the ethical conduct of doctors when dealing with dying patients.

POSTPONING DEATH: ABUSE OF CPR

One of the most troubling trends that has occurred in the practice of medicine in the modern North American hospital is a trap that many doctors and nurses have fallen into, and not always of their choosing. This is the trend towards treating every death as a cardiac arrest. Whether motivated by a desire to fight death to the bitter end or fear of being sued by the grieving family when the patient dies, many doctors don't seem to see that there is any difference between the forty-five-year-old woman in the final stages of terminal breast cancer that has spread to her bone and brain, the forty-five-year-old man who has just suffered his first heart attack, the eighty-two-year-old woman with Alzheimer's disease, and the six-year-old child who has fallen through the ice while skating and is suffering from profound hypothermia.

If you try to put yourself in the position of any of these patients, we are certain that you will see a difference from both a medical and a moral perspective. It has become easier for doctors to simply act first and ask questions later. This situation of not making a decision becomes an important decision all by itself. This approach is starting to draw fire from those who do, indeed, see the differences in these patients.

There are three important questions that doctors need to consider:

- Does CPR do any good for the patient?
- Does CPR protect the patient from any harm?
- Is this what the patient would want?

If the procedure is examined from a medical and social perspective and is found not to be good for the patient and not to protect him or her from harm, clearly it is a questionable decision. If the patient would not want it anyway, then, based on the belief in patient autonomy, the decision seems quite straightforward: the patient's wishes take precedence. If, on the other hand, it will be of no benefit, but the patient or the family asks for it anyway, what is the doctor to do? In light of the strained situation that health care faces today regarding resources, it seems immoral to undertake a procedure believed to be medically futile. Furthermore, it seems immoral for a family to put a doctor in this position. But a lack of clear understanding of the benefits and outcomes causes families to make these unreasonable requests anyway.

GIVING DEATH A HELPING HAND

Just begin a conversation about euthanasia at a gathering and watch the polarization of those taking part. Even if these people are all physicians, the movement to sides for and against will begin almost immediately. Euthanasia, or 'mercy killing' as it has been called, is an issue that is reaching the public agenda more and more frequently, and doctors themselves are intimately involved in these discussions and deeply divided about how it should be handled.

It is ironic that the word 'euthanasia,' which has its roots in the Greek for 'a good death,' should cause such division within the ranks of health professionals. Euthanasia comes in various forms, according to modern usage of the term. 'Active euthanasia,' where someone other than the dying person actually causes the death to happen, is differentiated from 'passive euthanasia,' which has been equated with following a dying person's wishes to withhold more life-sustaining treatment. Euthanasia is further divided into 'voluntary euthanasia' and 'involuntary euthanasia.' The former is, naturally, a situation in which the patient has specifically requested euthanasia, while the latter is a situation in which the individual was unable to consent and thus someone made such a decision for him or her. The natural extension of this would be for someone, perhaps a family member, to request euthanasia for a loved one, even if the person would be able to consent if he or she had been consulted. These are the occasions where someone else is deciding what is best for the dying person.

Clearly, there is no single answer to the question of how doctors approach the issue of euthanasia. A doctor who might favour voluntary, passive euthanasia as being morally acceptable may not feel the same way about his or her involvement in active euthanasia, and especially in involuntary euthanasia. Generally, doctors' opinions on these issues fall somewhere in the middle ground: the doctor may understand why a patient might wish to have his or her life ended, but may not want to take on the awesome responsibility involved in making such a value-laden decision. Add onto this the fact that their professional associations have not developed clear guidelines, and what remains to direct the choice is the law. Current legal standards make active euthanasia a criminal offence, giving doctors only legal guidance for a moral problem. Not everything that is moral is legal, and not everything that is legal is ethical.

In November 1991, the voters of Washington state defeated a law that would have made that state the only jurisdiction in North America to have legalized euthanasia. While 54 per cent of the population voted against the measure, what is interesting is that 46 per cent of those who voted (and the turnout included 62 per cent of eligible voters) supported it. The Washington

State Medical Association was among those who did not support the bill, insisting that it is the doctor's role to save lives, not cause deaths. In response to their stance, the medical association president, Dr James Kilduff, was quoted as saying, 'As physicians, our role is to provide care and compassion for terminal patients and that includes efforts to better educate the profession on pain management' (Fiscus and McMahon 1991, 10).

Most medical professional associations have not provided specific euthanasia guidelines for their members. Although most acknowledge that times are changing and moral values vary considerably, the general opinion is that it is unacceptable for a doctor to assist in ending a patient's life. While this is the generally publicised point of view, a study of doctors' attitudes and practices at the end of patients' lives, reported in 1991, indicated that almost 60 per cent of the responding doctors had been involved in disconnecting a patient's respirator, and almost 45 per cent had indirectly, but intentionally, assisted in a patient's death. This study did, however, have a somewhat small sample. The survey was mailed to 2,000 doctors, and 25 per cent responded (Kuznar 1991) – a poor response rate by anyone's standards.

In 1987, the World Medical Association approved a declaration that read, in part, 'Euthanasia ... even at the patient's own request or at the request of close relatives, is unethical.' While this speaks directly to the issue of active euthanasia, the statement goes on to indicate that the physician certainly can respect 'the desire of a patient to allow the natural process of death to follow its course in the terminal phase of sickness' (Williams and colleagues 1993, 1295). The American Medical Association, the Canadian Medical Association, and the British Medical Association have all taken similar stances. So it seems that the guidelines consider it unethical for doctors to practise active euthanasia, but ethical for doctors to be involved in passive euthanasia. Criticism can easily be levelled at the medical profession for deciding that it is more ethical to sit back and watch a patient suffer awaiting an inevitable death than it is to shorten that suffering.

There are, however, doctors who are troubled by what they

see as 'arbitrary, artificial lines' that these guidelines have drawn between the actual act of turning off a respirator, for example, and letting nature take its course, and hastening a death by an injection of morphine (Mullens 1993). Overall, doctors seem to want society to make the decision, and not leave it up to them.

The Royal Dutch Medical Association, however, has a slightly different perspective. They have taken the position that euthanasia belongs within the doctor–patient relationship, and that doctors, as a group, have a responsibility to ensure that public-policy arrangements are made so that this may be done. They have made it clear that, from their point of view, doctors are the only ones who should be involved in the practice.

Another issue that has divided both the public and doctors is the problem of 'assisted suicide.' Who among us has not heard of Derek Humphry's book *Final Exit: The Practicalities of Self-Deliverance and Assisted Suicide for the Dying*, which arrived on the bookshelves in 1991. When it was published, some people suggested that it should be banned, that it was encouraging people to take their lives. A young woman who killed herself in Montreal was found with the book at her side. Then, of course, there is the now-notorious Dr Kevorkian and his suicide machines. His well-intentioned approach to assisting people in voluntarily ending their lives has been criticized by many of his colleagues, but he continued his illegal activities because he believed he was doing the ethical thing. Recent legal challenges have resulted in his agreement to stop such activities.

In 1991, the results of a Canadian Gallup poll indicated that 75 per cent of Canadians agree or tend to agree with Dr Kevorkian and what he represents. They supported the notion that the laws should be changed so that terminally ill people who are suffering should have the right to have a doctor assist them in killing themselves. In general, doctors in both Canada and the United States clearly do not want to be the ones to give such help.

With all this apparent disagreement about what is right and ethical regarding our inevitable deaths, perhaps there are some things that are being done today in health care to rehumanize this increasingly sterile process.

PATIENTS IN CONTROL: THE ADVANCE DIRECTIVE

In 1990, there wasn't a media-savvy person in North America who didn't feel intimately involved in what should have been a private matter between a doctor and a patient. The legal battle it spawned was irresistible to the news media and gave us some insight into just how difficult it seems to maintain control over your own life and death. The patient was Nancy Cruzan, and the legal battle erupted over her parents' request for permission to end their thirty-two-year-old daughter's life.

Comatose since a car accident in 1983, Nancy Cruzan was severely brain damaged, but not 'brain dead' as we have come to define it. Her parents' request was based on the belief that quantity was not the appropriate yardstick with which to measure the quality of Nancy's life. The U.S. Supreme Court finally ruled that she could be allowed to die if there was *clear and convincing evidence that she would want to*. Although Nancy had not left a written document to indicate her wishes, a former co-worker testified that she had said that she would not want to live this way. The parents' request was granted, and her feeding tube was removed.

What this legal decision did was give credence to the notion that we have a moral and a legal right to make decisions for ourselves about our deaths, and that those decisions can be made long before we are ever faced with imminent death. What we are talking about here is what has come to be known as the 'living will.'

The living will was first given legal life in California in 1976, and since then the 1991 federal Patient Self-Determination Act in the United States requires that all patients be asked upon admission to hospital if they are aware of their right to refuse treatment and whether or not they have signed a living will. Several Canadian provinces have laws governing living wills, but they do not make it a mandatory part of health care in any way. While this is encouraging for those of us who would like to have some control over our own important decisions, how these documents are treated by doctors bears some examination.

If doctors are supposed to be so knowledgeable and ethical, why would they not make the right decisions for the patients – in other words, make decisions based on patients's wishes whether the patient has specified them or not? The fact is, doctors often don't know what the patient would have wanted. In a 1991 study of hospital outpatients reported in *Family Practice*, researchers found that 90 per cent wanted some kind of advance directive and that almost 80 per cent said that they wanted one because they feared excessive treatment by doctors. While we might want to think that these fears are not justified, the fact is that previous studies found that families, and especially doctors, were inaccurate in guessing what the patient would have wanted.

Even if a patient has a living will, doctors are not sure how they feel about them. During a 1992 ethics seminar in London, Ontario, one Canadian doctor who was the coordinator of an intensive care unit said that he didn't know how to satisfy himself that the patient really understood the implications of his or her actions when drawing up a living will (Johnston 1992). He would not know when to believe the patient. These attitudes make it very difficult for patients to maintain their autonomy.

In other studies doctors have indicated that they have positive attitudes towards living wills, but that they don't usually suggest that a patient should consider such a document. One study of doctors' and nurses' attitudes towards living wills found an important difference in opinion, depending upon the area of specialty. In this case, the researchers found that oncologists (specialists in cancer treatment) and intensive care specialists had the most reservations, while family doctors and those who specialize in the care of the elderly had the most positive attitudes towards living wills (Kelner and colleagues 1993).

The Canadian Medical Association has supplied its members with guidelines concerning living wills. These guidelines clearly tell doctors that, regardless of how they might feel about the constraints placed on them by the living will, the patient's wishes are to be followed. The guidelines further indicate that doctors should involve themselves in the development of these documents so that patients may understand exactly what their directives will mean in practice.

While doctors and patients will continue to disagree from time to time on how, when, and where it is appropriate to die, one thing is becoming clear: the 'life of any type, at any cost' attitude is sadly outdated, whether it comes from a physician or from a patient. We all need to take a closer look at what we should do to effect the dignity of the final chapter of our lives – our death.

18
The Ethics of the Future:
Patients Helping Doctors

At times the relationship between doctors (and patients) seems to
be founded on mutual distrust and disrespect. The awe is gone.
– Dr Paul Fink, Philadelphia, to Canadian Medical Association
Leadership Conference, 1993.

Dr Fink was expressing a sentiment that is widely held by doctors practising medicine in North America today. It has been
quite a long time now since our family doctors and consultants
fell off their pedestals, and that is secretly bemoaned by more
than one of them. The fact is, however, that many patients miss
it too. Although there seems to be no requiem for the lost awe,
there is a longing for the days when a visit to the doctor's office
seemed free from outside interference, and the healing relationship flourished. It would be ideal, however, if we could bring
both patient autonomy and trust of doctors back into that tar-
nished relationship, and add mutual respect. There may be a
way.

As we have looked at the issues over the course of this book,
you may have begun to feel that many are so complex that you
could not possibly have a contribution to make in their solution. You are wrong. The very fact that you are interested and
want to learn more makes you an ideal contributor to the solutions. Do medical professionals need and want your help?
Clearly, they need your help, and most agree that they want it.
Doctors, however, have a long-standing image of being arro-

gant. While we are not suggesting that all doctors are arrogant, there is a public perception that physicians, as a group, still believe themselves to be above the crowd. If there is one fact that is well learned from the public relations professionals of today it is this: *perception is reality.* For all those people who believe doctors are arrogant, it is true, whether this is an objective assessment or not.

In his address to the Harvard Medical School in 1977, the former editor of the *New England Journal of Medicine* spoke about this very issue: arrogance in medicine. He pointed out that any occupational group that uses highly complex technological approaches in both how they think and what they do can be accused of arrogance. This is, in part, a result of the fact that specialized knowledge and skills give them a secret to which other mortals are not privy.

Later in his speech, however, he points out that 90 per cent of the visits patients make to doctors are prompted by conditions that either will get better by themselves anyway or modern medicine can't do anything about (like the common cold). Since doctors seem to be able to make patients feel better most of the time, there must be something more to the encounter than technological intervention. He calls it reassurance: 'If the physician is to be effective in alleviating the patient's complaints by such intangible means, it follows that the patient has to believe in the physician, that he has confidence in his help and reassurance ... He needs, if the treatment is to succeed, a physician whom he invests with authoritative experience and competence. He needs a physician from whom he will accept some domination' (Ingelfinger 1980, 1509).

The relationship that you have with your doctor, then, seems crucial to the success or failure of your medical care and to the extent that the care will meet the highest ethical standards.

HELP FROM OUTSIDE: THE MEDICAL ETHICIST

Of all the new health professionals that have developed over the past decade or two, one of the most peculiar has to be the medical ethicist. The specialist in dealing with ethical dilemmas evolved from the difficulties that medical professionals were having in solving the problems for themselves.

What, exactly, is an ethicist? There isn't 'exactly' an answer. Another result of rapidly developing medical technology, medical ethicists are a modern invention. As the number of medical dilemmas rose, so too did the need for people with special knowledge of how to answer moral questions. Even Hippocrates would likely have found the permutations and combinations of morality presented by today's health care daunting.

Ethicists' educational backgrounds and professional experiences vary considerably, and their responsibilities within the current health care system vary as well. While a few have clinical backgrounds (doctors, perhaps, and a few nurses and social workers), some are clergy and lawyers, but most are philosophers. These are people who are trained, not in the science of medicine at all, but in the study of the philosophy of morality. Some work as an integral part of the health care team, while others simply consult from afar. Many hospitals seek out the services of the medical ethicist sometimes for no other reason than to avoid costly legal battles.

In a nutshell, the medical ethicist is a philosopher with expertise in ethical theory and a special interest in its application to medical issues and situations. Ethicist-professor Arthur Schafer has described an ethicist as a moral firefighter (Schafer 1986).

PROS AND CONS OF ETHICISTS

Whatever their backgrounds and responsibilities, medical ethicists have been subject to a number of criticisms. First, although they have expertise in ethics from a philosophical perspective, they do not have a monopoly on knowing what is right and what is wrong. Those without advanced academic credentials are equally capable of making valid judgments.

Second, they often have little understanding of the very real problems of being clinically responsible for a patient. The *hypothetical* case considered in a university's philosophy classroom does not always transfer easily to the *real* case experienced by the doctor and the patient.

Finally, they are not the ones who have to convey these sensitive decisions to the patients. When the ethics consultation is over, the physician is still left with the patient and the family to work through the reactions to the recommended course of action.

What, then, do they have to offer? From a patient's point of view, they offer another perspective on difficult moral issues. While this sort of consultation often results in more questions rather than more answers, these are questions that should be addressed. A good clinical ethicist has some understanding of both moral issues and what health care delivery is all about. A good clinical ethicist offers a well-organized, well-informed, thoughtful consideration of the issues. A good clinical ethicist can communicate well on a number of levels: with his or her peers, with the doctors, nurses, and other health professionals involved in patient care, and, most important, with you, the patient.

What the patient needs in these situations is a solid understanding of both the scientific/medical issues and the humanistic/moral issues. It is a rare health professional who has both.

MORALITY BY CONSENSUS

Another source of help for the patient caught in a moral dilemma related to health care is the hospital ethics committee. Even small hospitals located in areas that do not have the services of a medical ethicist will have an ethics committee.

The institutional ethics committee evolved out of a 1976 legal judgment in the United States which recommended the use of such a committee to confirm the prognosis of a comatose young woman. That young woman was Karen Ann Quinlan, and her family had requested the termination of life-support systems. Ethics committees throughout North America now provide both support for medical decisions and actual moral decision making for specific situations.

In addition to this role, however, the ethics committee in a hospital also has a role to play in educating health professionals about ethical issues and in making hospital policy. For that reason, the make-up of that committee is all-important.

One fact that doctors sometimes forget is that ethics in health care is not just ethics in medical care. The fact is that this is an interdisciplinary issue, and doctors are not the only professionals whose expertise helps patients to make decisions. Thus, these committees are generally made up of physicians, nurses, social workers, and clergy, but, given the increasingly technical and specialized nature of the environment of health care, technicians of all sorts, therapists, psychologists, pharmacists, and others could play valuable roles. Some ethics committees also have lay representatives from the community, and this is particularly useful for cultural representation. All members must be completely supportive of the roles and aims of the committee and willing to learn as much as possible about the ethics of health care.

This notion of making moral decision by group consensus is not confined to ethics committees in health care institutions. There is a growing movement across the continent for health care consumers to play an increasing role, and this movement has been called the 'Community Health Decisions' movement. The layperson is playing an increasingly important role in the development of bioethics policy, and the future of ethical judgments in health care rests with the community.

THE FUTURE

So long as I continue to be true to this Oath, may I be granted happiness of life, the practice of my art and the continuing respect of all men. But if I forswear and violate this Oath, may my fate be the opposite.

And so ends the Oath of Hippocrates. It seems that, if modern society could decide what it believed was right and wrong, and if all doctors knew this and adhered to a code of conduct that was unswerving, and we were all above being human, there might not be so many ethical dilemmas in medical care. The fact is, however, we are all fickle humans, and we all make mistakes.

Dr Goode wasn't certain what he had let himself in for when he agreed to sit on a public panel to discuss ethics in medicine. He was the representative of the primary-care doctor – the family physician. When he walked into the waiting-room behind the stage at the hotel where this televised meeting was to take place, the room was empty. He poured himself a cup of coffee and was just about to sit down when Dr Smart came in. He had met her briefly at a conference just last year and he wasn't certain she would remember him.

'Barry Goode, isn't it?' she said as she extended her hand. 'I'm Ursula Smart.'

'Nice to see you again,' he said as he shook her hand. 'You're here to give the perspective of the high-tech-medicine people, are you?'

'Yes,' she said as she sat down, 'but I'm no ethics expert. All I know is that there are hundreds of ethical issues that we confront daily and we do the best we can.'

Just then, a tall man with greying hair walked in and poured himself a cup of coffee. He turned towards where they were seated on the sofa. 'You must be my co-panelists. I'm Ian Wright. I'm the director of the bioethics institute at City University Medical School.'

Both Dr Goode and Dr Smart had heard his name before, but neither had met him.

'Well,' said Dr Smart, 'I guess you're the ethics expert. Glad to meet you.'

Dr Wright sat down opposite the sofa. 'Do you really think this is such a good idea? I mean, how many people out there in that audience, not to mention the media types who will be here, can really understand any of this?'

'I suppose that's why they invited us. It's our job to help them to understand,' said Dr Goode. 'I know I could use more help from my patients sometimes in giving them advice on ethically loaded problems.'

Dr Wright nodded. Just then the moderator of the panel appeared at the door and beckoned to them. 'There's one other panellist, but he'll join us on stage. Are you ready?'

They all got up and followed her out to the stage and took their places. When introductions were complete, the discussion began. In an hour, they covered issues ranging from the every-day problems in the family doctor's office, through the high drama of the intensive care units, to the help health care con-sumers can get from the medical ethicists. In the middle of it all was the fourth panellist, a patient. He represented all patients who have questions and confusions, and both want to be helped and to help.

Towards the end of the show, the moderator turned to the patient. 'Mr Blood, how do you think patients and doctors can help each other face these complex issues?'

Mr Blood sat thoughtfully for a second. 'I would say this to patients: Remember that the doctor is knowledgeable. Remem-ber that the doctor cares. Remember that the doctor is a person, not a god. I would say this to the doctor: Forget you're the doc-tor. Forget I'm a patient. Listen to me as a person.'

References

CHAPTER ONE

Baker, R., D. Porter, and R. Porter, eds. 1993. *The Codification of Medical Morality*. Boston: Kluwer Academic Publishers
Holmes, O. 1988. 'Practical Ethics of the Physician.' *Humane Medicine*, November, 129–30

CHAPTER TWO

Balkos, G. 1983. 'The Ethically Trained Physician: Myth or Reality?' *Canadian Medical Association Journal* 128, 682–4
Canadian Medical Association 1968. Minutes of the 1st Annual Meeting, 2–4 September, Montreal, Quebec
– 1990. *Code of Ethics*. Ottawa
Cousins, N. 1988. 'The Barracuda Syndrome.' *Humane Medicine*, November, 79–80
Inlander, C., L. Levin, and E. Weiner. 1988. *Medicine on Trial: The Appalling Story of Ineptitude, Malfeasance, Neglect and Arrogance*. Englewood Cliffs, NJ: Prentice-Hall
Kluge, E. 1992. Letter. *Canadian Medical Association Journal*, 147, 1234
Lynch, A. 1989. 'Symposium '89: Medical Ethics Education for the Undergraduate Medical Student.' *Westminster Affairs* 2 (Winter), 1–3
Pellegrino, E., R. Hart, S. Henderson, S. Loeb, and G. Edwards. 1985. 'Relevance and Utility of Courses in Medical Ethics: A Survey of Physicians' Perceptions.' *Journal of the American Medical Association* 253, 49–53

Pole, K. 1989. 'Why Is New Ethics Body So Unsure of Its Stance?' *Medical Post*, 7 February, 10

Rest, J. 1986. *Moral Development: Advances in Research and Theory.* New York: Praeger

Self, D., D.E. Schrader, D.C. Baldwin, Jr, and F.D. Wolinsky 1993. 'The Moral Development of Medical Students: A Pilot Study of the Possible Influence of Medical Education.' *Medical Education* 27/1, 26–34

Self, D., F. Wolinsky, and D. Baldwin. 1989. 'The Effect of Teaching Medical Ethics on Medical Students' Moral Reasoning.' *Academic Medicine* 64/12, 755–9

Tiberius, R., and D. Cleave-Hogg. 1984. 'Changes in Undergraduate Attitudes Toward Medical Ethics.' *Canadian Medical Association Journal* 130, 724–7

CHAPTER THREE

Devroede, G. 1991. 'A Surgeon's Reply.' *Humane Medicine* 7/1, 56–8

Gibbs, N. 1989. 'Sick and Tired.' *Time*, 31 July, 28–33

Ubelacker, S. 1993. 'Questioning the Doctor.' *Canadian Press Wire Service*, 6 January

CHAPTER FOUR

American Medical Association. 1980. *Principles of Medical Ethics.* Chicago

Annas, G. 1989. 'Privacy and Confidentiality,' In *The Rights of Patients: The Basic ACLU Guide*, 2d ed., 175–95. Carbondale and Edwardsville: Southern Illinois University Press

Canadian Medical Assocation. 1990. *Code of Ethics.* Ottawa

Goldberg, J. 1992. 'Who's Reading Your Medical Record?' *Lear's*, November, 40, 42

International code of medical ethics. 1983.

Norton, C. 1989. 'Absolutely Not Confidential.' *Hippocrates* 3/2, 52–60

Squires, B. 1992. 'Confidentiality and Research' (editorial). *Canadian Medical Association Journal* 147, 1299

CHAPTER FIVE

Biomedical Ethics Committee, Royal College of Physicians and Surgeons of Canada. 1987. *Informed Consent: Ethical Considerations for Physicians and Surgeons*

Cahn, C. 1980. 'Consent in Psychiatry: The Position of the Canadian Psychiatric Association.' *Canadian Journal of Psychiatry* 25, 78–85

Canadian Medical Association. 1986. 'CMA Policy on Informed Decision-Making.' *Canadian Medical Association Journal* 135, 1208A

Katz, J. 1992. 'Duty and Caring in the Age of Informed Consent and Medical Science: Unlocking Peabody's Secret.' *Humane Medicine* 8, 187–97

Silverman, W. 1989. 'The Myth of Informed Consent: In Daily Practice and Clinical Trials.' *Journal of Medical Ethics* 15, 6–11

CHAPTER SIX

Canadian Medical Association. 1868. *Code of Medical Ethics.* Appendix to the Minutes of the First Annual Meeting. Montreal

Dunn, K. 1992. 'Montreal M.D.'s AIDS-Related Collapse Raises Disclosure Issue at McGill Teaching Hospitals.' *Canadian Medical Association Journal* 147, 1362–4

Inlander, C., L. Levin, and E. Weiner. 1988. *Medicine on Trial: The Appalling Story of Ineptitude, Malfeasance, Neglect and Arrogance.* Englewood Cliffs, NJ: Prentice-Hall

Inlander, C., and E. Pavalon. 1990. *Your Medical Rights: How to Become an Empowered Consumer.* Boston: Little, Brown

McQueen, M. 1992. 'Conflicting Rights of Patients and Health Care Workers Exposed to Blood-Borne Infection.' *Canadian Medical Association Journal* 147, 299-302

Mayer, R. 1989. *The Consumer Movement: Guardians of the Marketplace.* Boston: Twayne

Morgan, B. 1993. 'Patient Access to MRI Centers in Orange County, California.' *New England Journal of Medicine* 328, 884–5

National Health Federation. 1970. Silver Anniversary Booklet

Sorenson, H. 1978. *The Consumer Movement.* New York: Arno Press

CHAPTER SEVEN

Fried, C. 1977. 'An Analysis of "Equality" and "Rights" in Medical Care.' *Nursing Digest* 5, 68–71

McCann, B. 1993. 'Kidney Disease Patients Face Gender, Age Bias.' *Family Practice* 5/5, 9

Morgan, B. 1993. 'Patient Access to MRI Centers in Orange County, California.' *New England Journal of Medicine* 328, 884–5

Parsons, A. 1985. 'Allocating Health Care Resources: A Moral Dilemma.' *Canadian Medical Association Journal* 132, 466–9

Rachlis, M., and C. Kushner. 1989. *Second Opinion: What's Wrong with Canada's Health Care System and How to Fix It.* Toronto: Collins

Ramsay, J. 1991. 'Hard Choices.' *Sunday Daily News,* 5 May, 16–17

Rooks, J. 1990. 'Let's Admit We Ration Health Care – Then Set Priorities.' *American Journal of Nursing* 90/6, 39–43

Smith, E. 1991. 'Allocation of Health Care Resources.' *Canadian Journal of Cardiology* 7, vi

Winslow, C., J.B. Kosecoff, M. Chassin, D.E. Kanouse, and R.H. Brook. 1988. 'The Appropriateness of Performing Coronary Artery Bypass Surgery.' *Journal of the American Medical Association* 260, 505–9

CHAPTER EIGHT

Arkinstall, W. 1993. Letter. *Canadian Medical Association Journal* 148, 485

Gullens, M. 1992. 'Doctors' Behaviour Influenced by Dealings with Drug Companies.' *Medical Post,* 17 November

Jablonsky, G. 1993. Letter. *Canadian Medical Association Journal* 148, 486

CHAPTER NINE

Huston, P. 1992. 'Is Health Technology Assessment Medicine's Rising Star?' *Canadian Medical Association Journal* 147, 1839–40

James, A.E., R.M. Zaner, J.E. Chapman, and C.L. Partain. 1990. 'Technology and Turf: Medicine in Conflict.' *Humane Medicine* 6/4, 264–8

Jecker, N. 1991. 'Knowing When to Stop: The Limits of Medicine.' *Hastings Center Report* 21/33, 5–8

Kucharesky, D. 1991. 'Be Proud of Our MI Therapy.' *Family Practice* 1, 16 November

Quivey, M. 1990. 'Advanced Medical Technology: Finding the Answers.' *International Nursing Review* 37, 329–30, 344

Rachlis, M., and C. Kushner. 1989. *Second Opinion: What's Wrong with Canada's Health Care System and How to Fix It.* Toronto: Collins

Technology Subcommittee of the Working Group on Critical Care, Ontario Ministry of Health. 1991. 'Guidelines for Medical Technology in Critical Care.' *Canadian Medical Association Journal* 144, 1617–22

'Wasted Health Care Dollars.' 1992. *Consumer Reports*, July, 435–48

CHAPTER TEN

Cohen, C. 1986. 'Can Autonomy and Equity Coexist in the ICU?' *Hastings Center Report* 16/5, 39–41

Hutchison, R. 1988. 'The "High-Tech Chronic": A New Kind of Patient.' *Humane Medicine* 4 (November), 118–19

Jennett, B. 1984. 'Inappropriate Use of Intensive Care.' *British Medical Journal* 289, 1709–11

Truog, R. 1992. 'Triage in the ICU.' *Hastings Center Report* 22/2, 13–17

CHAPTER ELEVEN

Bain, J. no date. 'Ethical Questions in Reproductive Medicine.' *In Ethics in Medical Practice*, 2–4. St. Laurent, PQ: Kommunicon Publications

Curie, M., and L. Cohen. 1979. 'Current Practice of Artificial Insemination by Donor in the United States.' *New England Journal of Medicine* 300, 585

'Doctor Found Guilty in Fertility Case.' 1992. *The New York Times*, 5 March, A, 14:1

Hill, E. 1986. 'Your Morality or Mine? An Inquiry into the Ethics of Human Reproduction – Presidential Address.' *American Journal of Obstetrics and Gynecology* 154, 1173–80

Rothschild, J. 1991. 'Engineering "the Perfect Child": Toward a New Hierarchy of Birth.' Paper presented at Mount Saint Vincent University, Halifax, NS, 17 January

Wallis, C. 1984. 'The New Origins of Life.' *Time*, 10 September, 40, 42–4, 49, 51

Wertz, D., and J. Fletcher. 1989. 'Fatal Knowledge? Prenatal Diagnosis and Sex Selection.' *Hastings Center Report* 19 (May-June), 21–7

CHAPTER TWELVE

Fost, N. 1981. 'Ethical Issues in the Treatment of Critically Ill Newborns.' *Pediatric Annals* 10, 383–8

O'Neill, J. 1983. 'Save Lives of Babies with Defects MD's Told.' *The Globe and Mail*, 30 November
Rostain, A., and V. Bhutani. 1989. 'Ethical Dilemmas of Neonatal-Perinatal Surgery.' *Clinics in Perinatology* 16/1, 275–302
Zupancic, J. 1992. 'Dangerous Economics: Resource Allocation in the NICU.' *Canadian Medical Association Journal* 146, 1073–6

CHAPTER THIRTEEN

'Abortions Should Be Manipulated for Fetal Tissue Harvest.' 1992. *Family Practice*, 5 October
Balk, R. 1990. 'Should Transplantation Be a Part of Our Health Care System?' *Canadian Family Physician* 36, 1129–32
Fox, R., and J. Swazey. 1992. 'Leaving the Field.' *Hastings Center Report* 22/5, 9–15
Hough, G. 1988. *News Writing*, 4th ed. Boston: Houghton Mifflin
Johnston, C. 1993. 'Transplanting Animal Organs into Humans Could Soon Become a Reality in Canada.' *The Medical Post*, 5 January 2
Kutner, N. 1987. 'Issues in the Application of High Cost Medical Technology: The Case of Organ Transplantation.' *Journal of Health and Social Behaviour* 28, 23–6
Paulette, L. 1993. 'A Choice for K'aila.' *Humane Medicine* 19 January, 13–17
'Possible Hearts for Donation Falling Through the Cracks, AHA Says.' 1992. *Family Practice*, 5 October, 6
Sutherland, R. 1993. 'Your Body! What an Investment!' *Family Practice*, 15 February, 23
Weber, S. 1992. 'Doctors Accept Use of Fetal Tissue ... in Theory.' *Medical Post*, 10 November, 48

CHAPTER FOURTEEN

Canadian Press. 1990. 'Medical Students Fear AIDS – Survey.' *The Halifax Herald*, 21 May
Dickey, N. 1989. 'Physicians and Immunodeficiency Syndrome: A Reply to Patients' (editorial). *Journal of the American Medical Association* 262, 2002
Gerbert, B., B. Maguire, S. Hulley, and T. Coates. 1989. 'Physicians and Acquired Immunodeficiency Syndrome.' *Journal of the American Medical Association* 262, 1969–72

Gilmore, N., and M. Somerville. 1989. 'Physicians, Ethics and AIDS: A Discussion Paper.' Ottawa: The Canadian Medical Association

Grady, C. 1989. 'Ethical Issues in Providing Nursing Care to Human Immunodeficiency Virus–Inflicted Populations.' *Nursing Clinics of North America* 24, 523–34

Gray, C. 1993. 'In the US, AIDS Has Become a "Marginal" Disease that Affects Thousands.' *Canadian Medical Association Journal* 148, 1369–73

Health and Welfare Canada. 1989. *AIDS: Everyone's Concern.* Ottawa: Supply and Services Canada

Kluge, E. 1991. 'Ethical Issues Concerning the HIV Status of Physicians and Patients.' *Canadian Medical Association Journal* 145, 518–19

Lambert, C. 1992. Letter. *Canadian Medical Association Journal* 147, 576–8

Lord, D. 1993. 'Cases of HIV-Positive Health Care Workers Spark Fear among Former UK Patients.' *The Medical Post*, 23 March

Parsons, A., and P. Parsons. 1990. *Health Care Ethics.* Toronto: Wall and Emerson

Rachlis, A. 1990. 'New Developments in the Diagnosis of HIV Infection.' *Canadian Journal of Diagnosis*, February, 61–79

Solomon, G., and C. Mead. 1987. 'Considerations in the Treatment of the Gay Patient with AIDS or ARC.' *Humane Medicine* 3/1, 10–19

Steben, M. 1992. 'Infected Health Care Workers Pose Little Threat.' *Family Practice*, 6 January

Taylor, P., and R. Mickleburgh. 1991. 'Dentists Strive to Calm Patients' Fear of AIDS.' *The Globe and Mail*, 17 April

CHAPTER FIFTEEN

Kreidie, A. 1993. 'Sexual Abuse Legislation Robs Doctors of Rights.' *The Medical Post*, 9 March, 6

Lowry, F. 1993. 'Fatal Distraction.' *Family Practice*, 15 March, 27, 32

Moore, I. 1992. 'Sex Abuse Report Can Be Positive.' *Family Practice*, 5 October

Quinn, M. 1993. 'Bawdy Language: Ontario Doctors Draw the Line.' *Family Practice*, 15 February, 1, 6

'Report on Sexual Abuse.' 1992. *Newsletter – Provincial Medical Board of Nova Scotia* 17/3

Rutter, P. 1986. *Sex in the Forbidden Zone.* Los Angeles: Jeremy P. Tarcher

CHAPTER SIXTEEN

Beck, M. 1990. 'The Geezer Boom.' *Newsweek Special Edition,* Winter/ Spring, 62–3, 66, 68
George, V., and A. Dundes. 1978. 'The Gomer: A Figure of American Hospital Folk Speech.' *Journal of American Folklore* 91, 568–81
Hutchison, R. 1988. 'The 'High-Tech Chronic': A New Kind of Patient.' *Humane Medicine* 4/2, 118–19
Jahnigen, D., and R. Schrier. 1986. 'The Doctor/Patient Relationship in Geriatric Care.' *Geriatric Clinics of North America* 2/3, 457–64
Jecker, N. 1991. 'Knowing When to Stop: The Limits of Medicine.' *Hastings Center Report* 21/3, 5–8
Lusky, R. 1986. 'Anticipating Needs of the US Aged in the 21st Century.' *Social Science and Medicine* 23, 1217–27

CHAPTER SEVENTEEN

Fiscus, J., and D. McMahon. 1991. 'Washington Voters Decide Against Legal Euthanasia.' *The Medical Post,* 19 November, 10
Johnston, C. 1992. 'Living Wills Should Be Treated with Caution, ICU Director Tells Conference.' *Canadian Medical Association Journal* 147, 1370–1
Kelner, M., I. Bourgeault, P. Hébert, and F. Dunn. 1993. 'Advance Directives: The Views of Health Professionals.' *Canadian Medical Association Journal* 148, 1331–7
Kuznar, W. 1991. 'When It's Time to Die: Survey Reveals Physicians' Struggle with Ethics, the Law.' *Modern Medicine* 59 (July), 18, 20
Mullens, A. 1993. 'Society Must Lead in Determining Canadian Position on Euthanasia, Doctors Say.' *Canadian Medical Association Journal* 148, 1363, 1366–8
Williams, J., 1993. 'Canadian Physicians and Euthanasia: 1. An Approach to the Issue.' *Canadian Medical Association Journal* 148, 1293–7

CHAPTER EIGHTEEN

Ingelfinger, F. 1980. 'Arrogance.' *New England Journal of Medicine* 303, 1507–11
Schafer, A. 1986. 'Are Hospital Ethicists Doing a Worthwhile Job?' *The Globe and Mail,* 9 December, A7

Index

abortion: acceptability of to Medical Research Council of Canada, 131; as a form of contraception, 126; ethics and, 9, 131; fetal tissue transplantation and, 151; reproductive technology and, 126; selective, 128

Acer, David, and the transmission of AIDS, 75

ageing patients, 176–84; and ageism, 85, 177–84; and autonomy, 182; characterization of as GOMERs, 176; common diseases of, 180; confidentiality accorded to, 182–3; ethical dilemmas regarding, 181–3; life expectancy of, 179; organ transplantation and, 178; quality of life of, 180–1; relationship of with doctor, 183–4; resource allocation and, 84–5, 183

AIDS, 159–69; activists groups, 164–5; and Canadian Medical Association code of ethics, 164, 167; as a social issue, 161–2; definition of, 160–1; doctors' attitudes towards those with, 162–3; doctors' rights/patients' rights in relation to, 167–8; Health and Welfare Canada brochure on, 160; legal reporting of information on patients with, 23, 44–5, 48; mandatory testing for, 161, 163–5; media coverage of, 159–72, 164; and medical confidentiality, 74–6, 165–6; public opinion in relation to, 163–4; refusal to treat patients with, 22, 166–7; resource allocation for, 169; San Francisco Biopsychosocial AIDS Project, 163; U.S. Centers for Disease Control and, 168

allied health professionals, 37, 43, 112–13, 168; confidentiality and, 43, 46–7; ethics and, 201; health educators, 37; HIV infection and, 138; impact of,